Praise for
Individualized Autism Intervention for Young Children

"Deeply rooted in 50 years of research and practice, this book sets a new standard for being at once highly accessible, comprehensive, evidence based, and—with its emphasis on a blended intervention approach—*truly groundbreaking.* If you read one book on autism treatment, this should be it."

—Steven F. Warren, Ph.D.
Schiefelbusch Institute for Life Span Studies, University of Kansas, Lawrence

"Has immediate value . . . makes selecting the right methods for each child of prime importance. Thompson points the way toward a potentially fruitful approach for matching learners to teaching methods."

—Sandra L. Harris, Ph.D.
Douglass Developmental Disabilities Center, Rutgers,
The State University of New Jersey

"Travis Thompson brings a uniquely lucid voice into the jumbled world of behavioral interventions. His perspectives, emanating from deep experience as a scientist and as a family member, have produced a very sensible and useful guidebook grounded in the essential principle of individualization. Parents, clinicians, behavior analysts, and educators of all types will find great value in this book."

—Glen Dunlap, Ph.D.
University of South Florida

"Dr. Thompson is an amazing altruistic man and clinician. His ability to see the 'forest through the trees' has served us well and countless others, I am quite sure. As no two kids on the spectrum are the same, it would behoove clinicians, researchers, educators, and parents to match their therapeutic strategies to best match their children's needs. Dr. Thompson's work has exemplified this in practice and now through the power of books. Read and learn from a true master."

—Matthew Segedy, M.D.
Pediatrician and father of a daughter with autism

"The emphasis on combining highly structured teaching opportunities with teaching activities that are embedded in naturally occurring situations is a welcomed approach for parents and professionals alike. Dr. Thompson and his colleagues are applauded for encouraging individualized decision making and outcome assessment to maximize functional skill development that contributes to a child's ultimate success."

—Dawn Buffington Townsend, Ph.D., BCBA-D
Institute for Educational Achievement

"I will be purchasing this book and will definitely be recommending it. . . . Dr. Thompson has done an excellent job documenting the research and covering most questions, concerns, and issues [surrounding selection of] the most effective and efficient approach for each unique child."

—Dr. Suzanne Jacobsen, R.Psych., BCBA-D
Clinical Director, ABA Learning Centre, Richmond, BC, Canada

"Highlights the hope in individualizing autism interventions and illustrates how that process can yield better results for our children. I applaud Dr. Thompson for writing about this complex approach, one that challenges us to modernize how we view and treat ASD, and therefore, stands to benefit all who are affected by it."

—Cindy Tupy
Mother of Lilly, who has Asperger syndrome

"With new data showing that nearly half of children diagnosed on the Autism Spectrum will reach best outcomes with Early Intensive Behavioral Intervention, Dr. Thompson's data-driven resource for selecting treatment, interventions, and goals is an essential manual for parents and professionals. [Dr. Thompson] makes the data behind intervention and treatment accessible, enabling parents and professionals to make decisions scientifically supported to achieve best outcomes. [The] book carries you through the process of diagnosis and gives a new, more informed perspective on choosing the right combination of treatments."

—Tracy Reid, J.D.
Attorney, Cooper & Reid, LLC, and mother of a child with autism,
Minneapolis, Minnesota

Individualized
Autism
Intervention
for Young Children

Individualized Autism Intervention

for Young Children

Blending Discrete Trial and Naturalistic Strategies

by

Travis Thompson, Ph.D.
University of Minnesota
Minneapolis

with invited contributors

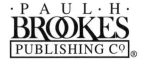

·P·A·U·L·H·
BROOKES
PUBLISHING C⁰ ®

Baltimore · London · Sydney

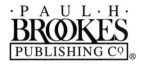

Paul H. Brookes Publishing Co.
Post Office Box 10624
Baltimore, Maryland 21285-0624
USA

www.brookespublishing.com

Typeset by Auburn Associates, Inc., Baltimore, Maryland.
Manufactured in the United States of America by
Sheridan Books, Inc., Chelsea, Michigan.

Cover photo of Patrick Ward by Clover A. Anderson and all other photos used by permission.

The individuals described in this book are composites or real people whose situations are masked when necessary and are based on the authors' experiences. In some instances, names and identifying details have been changed to protect confidentiality.

Library of Congress Cataloging-in-Publication Data

Thompson, Travis.
   Individualized autism intervention for young children: blending discrete trial and naturalistic strategies
/ by Travis Thompson.
      p.   cm.
   Includes bibliographical references and index.
   ISBN-13:   978-1-59857-173-8 (pbk.)
   ISBN-10:   1-59857-173-7 (pbk.)
   1. Autism in children.   2. Behavior therapy for children.   I. Title.
   RJ506.A9T46 2011
   618.92'85882—dc22   2011006539

British Library Cataloguing in Publication data are available from the British Library.

2015   2014   2013   2012   2011

10   9   8   7   6   5   4   3   2   1

Contents

About the Author

Travis Thompson, Ph.D., L.P., Graduate Faculty Member, Special Education Program, Department of Educational Psychology, University of Minnesota, Minneapolis, and Consulting Psychologist, Minnesota Early Autism Project, 7242 Forestview Lane North, Maple Grove, Minnesota 55369

Dr. Thompson is affiliated with the Autism Certificate Program in the Special Education Program of the Department of Educational Psychology at the University of Minnesota, and he is Adjunct Professor in the Department of Applied Behavioral Science at the University of Kansas, Lawrence. He is a collaborator on a multisite project on challenging behavior in developmental disabilities including the Kennedy Krieger Institute in Maryland; the Eunice Kennedy Shriver Center, University of Massachusetts, Amherst; and the University of Kansas, Parsons. He is a licensed psychologist. Dr. Thompson completed his doctoral training in psychology at the University of Minnesota and completed postdoctoral work at the University of Maryland. He spent a year at Cambridge University in the United Kingdom and a year as a visiting scientist at the National Institute on Drug Abuse in Rockville, Maryland. Dr. Thompson was Director of the John F. Kennedy Center for Research on Human Development at Vanderbilt University and Director of the Institute for Child Development at the University of Kansas Medical Center—a clinical, training, and research institute. Dr. Thompson has served on several National Institutes of Health research review committees, including chairing reviews of the applicants for Collaborative Programs of Excellence in Autism awards in 2000, 2003, and 2007. He has been a member of American Psychological Association (APA) task forces concerned with the practice of psychology and psychopharmacology. He is a past president of the Behavioral Pharmacology Society, the Division of Psychopharmacology and Substance Abuse, and the Division of Mental Retardation and Developmental Disabilities of the APA. Dr. Thompson has received numerous awards, including the Distinguished Research Award, The Arc of the United States; the Academy on Mental Retardation Lifetime Research Award; the APA's Don Hake Award; the Edgar A. Doll Award, for contributions to facilitate the transfer of research into practice; and the Ernest R. Hilgard Award and the Impact of Science on Application Award of the Society for Advancement of Behavior Analysis. He has served as cochair of the Association for Behavior Analysis International's Annual Autism Conference (2010 and 2011). He has published more than 230 journal articles and chapters and 30 books dealing with autism, developmental disabilities, psychopharmacology, and related topics. His most recent books, *Making Sense of Autism* (2007) and *Dr. Thompson's Straight Talk on Autism* (2008), are also published by Paul H. Brookes Publishing Co. Dr. Thompson has spoken in 46 states and 15 countries about his research and clinical services and on topics related to autism and other developmental disabilities and psychopharmacology.

About the Contributors

Clover A. Anderson, M.Ed., Advanced Senior Therapist, Minnesota Early Autism Project, 7242 Forestview Lane North, Maple Grove, Minnesota 55369

Ms. Anderson has been a professional in the field of early intervention and autism since the mid-1990s. Her professional life became personal when her son was diagnosed with autism at 19 months of age. She has taken that experience and devoted herself to providing effective and comprehensive treatment to children and families affected by autism.

Lisa M. Barsness, M.S., Clinic Director, Minnesota Early Autism Project, 7242 Forestview Lane North, Maple Grove, Minnesota 55369

Ms. Barsness completed her undergraduate training at the University of Wisconsin-Madison and her master's degree in applied behavior analysis at Saint Cloud State University in Minnesota. She has 16 years of experience providing Early Intensive Behavioral Treatment in both Wisconsin and Minnesota and has conducted numerous workshops across the United States, Canada, and England. In 2005, Lisa cofounded the Minnesota Early Autism Project with Glen Sallows, Tammlyn Sallows, and Travis Thompson.

Amy Bohannan, M.S., Board Certified Behavior Analyst, Minnesota Early Autism Project, 7242 Forestview Lane North, Maple Grove, Minnesota 55369

Ms. Bohannan has been working with children with autism since 1994 providing applied behavior analysis (ABA) services throughout the Midwest. She has been a supervisor at Minnesota Early Autism Project, providing Early Intensive Behavior Intervention to children with autism. She has also provided ABA services to school-age children and adolescents in home, community, and residential services with a variety of developmental disabilities.

Beth Burggraff, M.S., BCBA, Clinical Director, Minnesota Early Autism Project, (MEAP) 7242 Forestview Lane North, Maple Grove, Minnesota 55369

Ms. Burggraff received her undergraduate degree from the University of St. Thomas in elementary education/psychology and her graduate degree from St. Cloud State University in applied behavior analysis. She is also a Board Certified Behavior Analyst. Burggraff worked as a private behavior therapist for 5 years before taking a position as a senior behavior therapist with another Minnesota autism agency. From 2004–2006, she served as a director/clinical supervisor at the Minnesota Autism Center. She also worked in Chicago as a behavior analyst and department leader, serving children with autism spectrum disorders, attention-deficit/hyperactivity disorder, and behavioral concerns. In addition to serving as Clinical Director of MEAP, she is currently a treatment supervisor, providing Early Intensive Behavior Intervention to children with autism.

Patti L. Dropik, M.A., Advanced Senior Behavior Therapist, Minnesota Early Autism Project, 7242 Forestview Lane North, Maple Grove, Minnesota 55369

Ms. Dropik has been working with young children with autism spectrum disorders (ASDs) and other communication disorders since the mid-1990s. Currently, she develops and supervises home-based Early Intensive Behavioral Treatment programs for young children with ASDs. Her training in developmental and behavioral psychology together with her graduate studies in speech language pathology have fostered her focus in developing naturalistic teaching interventions for children with ASDs.

Foreword

Following on the heels of one of the most informative books for families about autism spectrum disorders (ASDs)—titled *Dr. Thompson's Straight Talk About Autism*—author Travis Thompson has returned to the role of scientist translator for families, and thus fills a much-needed role. Scientific reports on ASD and intervention practices are usually written for other scientists to read, and unless parents are themselves scientists, the information in research studies is not very interpretable. In this book Dr. Thompson describes in an understandable style what science tells us about the complexities, complications, and forms of ASDs as they relate to the selection and use of evidence-based intervention practices. A clear theme throughout the book is that ASD takes many forms, and the characteristics of individual children with ASDs should guide the therapist, teacher, and parent in selecting the intervention that will be the most appropriate. Achieving this match between a child and the intervention is complicated and not always intuitive. For parents who may still be reeling from their child's initial diagnosis or, alternatively, who may be reeling from having tried a second or third "sure-fire" therapy without results, locating the program that works for their child is at the forefront of their minds. This book will fill the parents' need for information about autism.

In his early chapters, Dr. Thompson provides the essential introductory information about the history and nature of autism and its evolution, as a concept and diagnosis, into ASD. Viewing autism as a "spectrum" disorder is a confusing notion for parents—and for practitioners and scientists. As Dr. Thompson explains, there are "disorders" (e.g., Asperger syndrome) that share similar characteristics with the formal Autistic Disorder specified by the American Psychiatric Association (APA; 2000) in their diagnostic manual but that differ on some specific features. The emerging consensus is that the similarities (shared characteristics of poor communication and social skills and repetitive behaviors) are greater than the differences among the associated diagnoses. Two practical implications exist for families. First, professionals may not always agree on which diagnosis applies to a child (i.e., the reliability of differential diagnosis is questionable), so family members may receive different diagnoses from different professionals. Second, if a child receives a diagnosis other then Autistic Disorder, he or she may be judged ineligible for services.

The APA is in the process of revising its diagnostic criteria, and in the next edition of this book, Dr. Thompson will probably report that the formal diagnostic term has been broadened to *Autism Spectrum Disorder*. The term is used often and somewhat inconsistently today but has not been formalized in the manuals and criteria that govern medical diagnoses. The current plans, still in formulation, are that the characteristics or expressions of ASD will vary along a range of severity—a spectrum. Using the color spectrum as a metaphor, one can imagine the color red ranging from intense dark red at one end to a very light pink at the other. Autism is seen as a spectrum disorder because it varies from severe to mild in its expression across individuals.

In this book, however, Dr. Thompson describes the details and complexities of ASD that go beyond the spectrum analogy and are critically important for parents to understand. That is, along with the social, communication, and behavioral concerns that are the defining elements of ASD, some children may experience intellectual disability, attention-deficit/hyperactive disorder, anxiety disorder, oppositional disorder, sleep disorder, or seizure disorder (in adolescence). The "or" in this sentence is important for parents to understand because children with ASD do not experience all of these bleak-sounding accompanying characteristics. But, they happen often enough for parents to be aware of the possibilities, and when planning intervention and services for children, it is critical to understand which accompanying characteristics exist.

Lest this paint too dark of a picture of ASD for parents, there is good news. As Dr. Thompson notes, there are characteristics of children and services that are predictors of positive responses to intervention. That is, if these characteristics occur, intervention approaches are more likely to produce positive results than if they are not present. Beginning intervention 1) early and 2) as intensively as possible are two important factors. Starting intervention in later childhood does not doom a child to a poor outcome, but the prospects are better if we start early. Also, Dr. Thompson makes the very important point that the strongest effects for intervention are in the first year or so of service, a point confirmed by others who have investigated different interventions (Dawson et al., 2009). So the plan to "ease into intervention and see how the child does" is not a good idea because it does not take advantage of the initial intervention impact.

Individual characteristics of children are also predictors of positive outcomes for children, and Dr. Thompson highlights several. Social interest and responsiveness, joint attention, social referencing, imitation, and use of words to communicate by the age of 5 are often identified as characteristics that suggest children will respond to intervention approaches. Of note, if a child does not have these characteristics, it does not doom them to poor outcomes. These predictors can become the focus or goals of very early interventions. For example, in our work with toddlers with ASD and their families, we have focused on promoting joint attention (Schertz & Odom, 2007; Schertz, Odom, & Baggett, 2010); with the rationale that joint attention will lead to more advanced communication and social abilities.

Evidence-based practice (EBP) is the watchword for the selection of intervention strategies for children with ASD and their families. Dr. Thompson describes well the roots of EBP in the evidence-based medicine movement that came across the pond from the United Kingdom. In the United States, there have been considerable efforts to identify interventions or "treatments" for which there is scientific evidence of effectiveness (National Autism Center, 2009; National Professional Development Center on Autism Spectrum Disorders, 2010). This is particularly important for children with ASD and their families because, as Dr. Thompson and others (Shute, 2010) note, researchers and purveyors have proposed many different treatments as effective when no evidence or contradictory evidence exists. Remember, at one time in the history of autism, the most informed scientific *opinion* was that "refrigerator mothers" caused autism and an acceptable treatment was a "parentecomy" (i.e., removing the parent from the child). As recently as the last 5 years, an acceptable practice in Europe (i.e., called packing) was to wrap children with ASD who had challenging behaviors in cold, wet blankets until they calmed (Spinney, 2007). In the United States, treatments without evidence are abundant (e.g., facilitated communication, diets, hyperbaric oxygen chambers). Even such traditional and often-used treatments as sensory integration, auditory integration, and such well-known comprehensive treatment programs such as Relationship Development Intervention or DIR (Floortime) have limited or weak published scientific support for their effects. Dr. Thompson explains well the concept of the placebo effect, which may account for positive testimonials that are sometimes offered in support of practices without scientific evidence.

To their credit, Dr. Thompson and his colleagues at the Minnesota Early Autism Project have built a program of intervention for children with ASD and their families on the most current research on effective interventions. As the reader will see, the intervention model is seated solidly in an applied behavioral analysis theoretical framework. While acknowledging the theoretical bases for a range of early childhood programs, he provides a strong rationale for the specific practices that make up the program. The elements of his program are supported by recent reviews of evidence-based, focused intervention practices and comprehensive treatment models for children with ASD (National Autism Center, 2009; Odom, Boyd, Hall, & Hume, 2010; Odom, Collet-Klingenberg, Rogers, & Hatton, 2010). Purists in the autism intervention field may view Dr. Thompson's program as eclectic (i.e., which is not used in a positive way here) because 1) it selects from a range of focused intervention practices in building an individualized program for young children and 2) it provides a comprehensive model of intervention, but it does not follow precisely an established and recognized comprehensive treatment model (e.g., the UCLA Young Autism Project, Pivotal Response Treatment, LEAP, TEACCH). This view would be shortsighted.

Elements of the early intervention model proposed by Dr. Thompson and implemented through the Minnesota Autism Intervention Program are built very solidly on a strong research base and enacted through the clinical wisdom that only comes with years of practice. Here are but a few critical elements of the program that Dr. Thompson describes.

· The child's individual characteristics drive the selection of intervention approaches employed. Dr. Thompson and colleagues have created a process for assessing children's initial skills and abilities and selecting the structure and intensity of the intervention approaches.

· Clinicians use a nationally known assessment, the Assessment of Basic Language and Learning Skills–Revised (Partington, 2007), to gather future information about the content of the intervention program.

· For children with severe and moderate levels of ASD, the program begins with a highly intense, Discrete Trial Intervention approach, which has strong support from the empirical literature.

· As children severely and moderately affected by ASD make progress in Discrete Trial Intervention, naturalistic (less structured) intervention is introduced. These approaches also have strong support from the literature.

· For children with milder expressions of ASD, naturalistic intervention approaches may be employed at the beginning of treatment.

These elements, assessment→intense structured intervention for a period of time→less structured intervention, very much characterize the current state of the art of the field. For example, the classic DTI model first developed by Ivar Lovaas (1987) has evolved into a model currently proposed by the Lovaas Institute (http://www.lovaas .com) that moves from Discrete Trial training to more naturalistic instruction. This process also extends across conceptual/theoretical orientations. The Early Start Denver Model (Rogers & Dawson, 2010), which operates from a developmental orientation, begins its intervention with children and families through intense, individualized, clinic-based intervention that sometimes includes Discrete Trial training and moves to more naturalistic strategies as children learn and develop. Progress, however, happens for many but not all children. For some, continued intensive DTI may be necessary, but the value of beginning early is that the impact for many will lead to less intense services down the line.

A particularly appealing feature of this book, in addition to its solid basis on research and science, is the frequent presentation of case studies. There is a danger in basing practice solely on stories, case studies, or one individual's clinical experience. But, when the stories elaborate approaches based in science, they bring the highly academic, rigorous, and methodologically heavy articles to life. In addition, the personal nature of the stories that Dr. Thompson brings to his writing instills confidence in the author. It is clear that this is not a person who sits in his office or watches through an observation window. In this book, Dr. Thompson speaks from science, experience, and the heart—a worthy combination.

In conclusion, this book draws together well the worlds of research and practice. Dr. Thompson provides current, basic information about ASD as a foundation for describing the process for building intervention programs that address the individuals needs of the child. The approaches he describes are very much in step with evidence-based, focused intervention practices and comprehensive treatment programs that are at the forefront of the field today. Family members and professionals will learn much from this book.

Samuel L. Odom, Ph.D.
Director, Frank Porter Graham Child Development Institute
University of North Carolina at Chapel Hill

REFERENCES

American Psychiatric Association. (2000). *Diagnostic and statistical manual of mental disorders* (4th ed., text rev.). Washington, DC: Author.

Dawson, G., Rogers, S., Munson, J., Smith, M., Winter, J., Greenson, J., et al. (2009). Randomized, controlled trial of an intervention for toddlers with autism: The Early Start Denver Model. *Pediatrics, 125*(1), e17–e23.

Lovaas, O.I. (1987). Behavioral treatment and normal educational and intellectual functioning in young autistic children. *Journal of Consulting and Clinical Psychology, 55*, 3–9.

National Autism Center. (2009). *National Standards Project: Findings and conclusions.* Randolph, MA. Retrieved December 16, 2010, from http://www.nationalautismcenter.org/pdf/NAC%20Findings%20&%20Conclusions.pdf

National Professional Development Center on Autism Spectrum Disorders. (2010). *Evidence-based practices.* Chapel Hill, NC: FPG Child Development Institute. Retrieved December 16, 2010, from http://autismpdc.fpg.unc.edu/content/evidence-based-practices

Odom, S.L., Boyd, B., Hall, L., & Hume, K. (2010). Evaluation of comprehensive treatment models for individuals with Autism Spectrum Disorders. *Journal of Autism and Developmental Disorders, 40*, 425–436.

Odom, S.L., Collet-Klingenberg, L., Rogers, S., & Hatton, D. (2010). Evidence-based practices for children and youth with Autism Spectrum Disorders. *Preventing School Failure, 54*, 275–282.

Partington, J. (2007). *ABLLS-R: The Assessment of Basic Language and Learning Skills–Revised.* Walnut Creek, CA. The Behavior Analysts, Inc.

Rogers, S.J., & Dawson, G. (2010). *Early Start Denver Model for young children with autism: Promoting language, learning, and engagement.* New York: Guilford Press.

Schertz, H.H., & Odom, S.L. (2007). Promoting joint attention in toddlers with autism: A parent-mediated approach. *Journal of Autism and Developmental Disorders, 37*, 1562–1575.

Schertz, H.H., Odom, S.L., & Baggett, C. (2010, October). *Intervention for toddlers with autism: The Joint Attention Mediated Learning Model.* Presentation at 26th Annual International Conference on Young Children with Special Needs and their families, Kansas City, MO.

Shute, N. (2010, October). Desperate for an autism cure. *Scientific American,* 80–85.

Spinney, L. (2007). Therapy for autistic children causes an outcry in France. *Lancet, 370*(9558), 645–646.

Thompson, T. (2008). *Dr. Thompson's straight talk about autism: The expert guide parents can trust.* Baltimore: Paul H. Brookes Publishing Co.

Preface

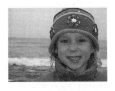

A parent of one of the children with autism with whom we are working (see photo at left) referred to me as "the autism whisperer," which I took to be a somewhat embarrassing, well-intentioned compliment. While I greatly appreciated this mother's sentiment, I don't think she was suggesting that there was any wizardry involved in my work with her child. I suspect she meant that, along with the staff of the Minnesota Early Autism Project, where I had been working, I was able to see the world through the eyes of her 4-year-old daughter with Autistic Disorder. As a result, it has been possible to individualize treatment that uniquely fit her needs. We used combinations of evidence-based methods that best fit the individual child, which is why I call the approach Blended Intervention.

We combine elements of Pivotal Response Treatment (Koegel & Koegel, 2006), Milieu Language Teaching (Kaiser & Hester, 1994), Incidental Teaching (Hart & Risley, 1975), and activity-based early intervention (Pretti-Frontczak & Bricker, 2004) with Discrete Trial Intervention (DTI; Lovaas, 1987) in various proportions, depending on a child's needs.

Over the past year, this woman's child, who had received largely DTI in the beginning, improved notably. Unlike Cesar Millan, the man known as "The Dog Whisperer" (Millan & Peltier, 2007), whom I imagine she had in mind with her comment, I have a great deal more in common with the children with whom I work than with Mr. Millan with his four-legged clients. When I observe a child with autism struggling to make sense of the world around her or him, I see the mixture of confusion, anxiety, and frustration on the child's face. I readily empathize with the child's dilemma.

A significant problem we face in the field of early autism services is that, too often, a child with autism is expected to fit within a service model rather than the model needing to fit the child. Parents are presented with a *potpourri* of service options from which to choose but find it difficult to sort out the conflicting information and claims. Proponents of each autism intervention model are convinced that theirs is the best approach for most, if not all, children with autism spectrum disorders. The result is confusion among parents, teachers, and policy makers, who strive to make sense of competing assertions. Efforts to determine a priori which treatment method will be most effective for a specific child is in its infancy (Stahmer, Schreibman, & Cunningham, 2010). This book suggests a concrete way of beginning to address this critical issue.

The field of reading instruction went through a similar period of turmoil in the 1980s and 1990s, when teachers chose between warring factions: those who advocated whole language approaches versus those who advocated phonics approaches. The whole language or literacy approach was largely the main educational reading strategy of the 1980s and until the mid-1990s. Despite its popularity during this period, educators who believed that focused skill instruction was important for students' learning and many educational researchers were skeptical of whole language claims. The 1990s saw significant declines in student achievement nationwide on the National Assessment of Educational Progress. Much of the blame for these declines was assigned to the emphasis on whole language reading instruction. Subsequent research indicates that while reading instruction in which phonics is taught explicitly is an essential educational strategy for most early readers, for some students it can be effectively supplemented using an approach in which phonics is taught incidentally, as in whole language approaches. However, blended approaches that integrate reading comprehension and writing with explicit instruction in phonics seem most effective, and supersede this decades-old conflict (Rayner, Foorman, Perfetti, Pesetsky, & Seidenberg, 2001; Stuebing, Barth, Cirino, Francis, & Fletcher, 2008). The degree of emphasis on different components can be tailored to different students helping teachers differentiate instruction in response to student progress, a more contemporary emphasis in reading instruction superseding the whole language versus phonics dichotomy.

My book, *Dr. Thompson's Straight Talk on Autism* (2007), was an attempt to present a practical, evidence-based approach to autism intervention for parents, teachers, and therapists, employing Discrete Trial Behavioral Interventions in combination with positive behavior support and cognitive behavioral approaches. That was a useful step in the right direction, but we have more work to do. The new book presents a case for individualized interventions for young children with autism spectrum disorders (ASDs), integrating elements from the University of California, Los Angeles (UCLA), Young Autism Discrete Trial Intervention with naturalistic interventions based on behavioral learning principles combined with activity-based early education. Although the strongest evidence from controlled studies supports the UCLA Young Autism DTI among comprehensive treatments, there are numerous studies indicating *components* of Pivotal Response Training, TEACCH, and at least one study indicating the Early Start Denver Model (Dawson et al., 2009) can be effective as well. At the Minnesota Early Autism Project, a home-based, intensive early behavioral intervention service, approximately half of the children with whom we work receive combined intervention strategies, and roughly one quarter each receive a largely Discrete Trial or largely Incidental Intervention approach. Our outcome data, discussed briefly in the postscript, are encouraging, with all but about 10% achieving significant improvements in intellectual, language, and social functioning, as well as reductions in emotional-behavioral features of autism.

Choice of intervention approach is substantially based on an understanding of the nature of—and variability in—expression of autism symptoms. Chapter 1 discusses changes that have occurred in our understanding of autism, including recent information about autism subtypes. Autism can be best understood as a dimensional disability and through degrees of manifestation of core features and factors that moderate their expression (Chapter 2). Questions are often raised about whether autism is a unique disability because it often overlaps with other conditions, which are explored in Chapter 3. One of the more important sections in the book, Chapter 4, examines predictors of a child's response to intervention. Although there has been a great deal of discussion of effectiveness of specific intervention methods, little attention has been paid to child factors affecting outcome, which are also examined in Chapter 4. Chapter 5 discusses evidence-based practice and what that means. The goal is to match interventions that are based on solid evidence with child characteristics. Chapter 6 explores intervention dimensions of similarities and differences across interventions that appear to be very different from one another. Sometimes there are important similarities in otherwise dissimilar models.

Section II of the book presents guiding principles and practical methods for illustrative interventions ranging from Discrete Trial Intervention (Chapter 7) to Incidental Teaching (Chapter 8) and blended combinations of each (Chapters 9 and 10). The postscript discusses preliminary outcomes of our work with a Blended Intervention approach and explores rapid emergence of promising new knowledge in autism research.

REFERENCES

Dawson, G., Rogers, S., Munson, J., Smith, M., Winter, J., Greenson, J., et al. (2009). Randomized, controlled trial of an intervention for toddlers with autism: The Early Start Denver Model. *Pediatrics, 125*(1), e17–e23.

Hart, B., & Risley, T.R. (1975). Incidental teaching of language in the preschool. *Journal of Applied Behavior Analysis, 8,* 411–420.

Kaiser, A.P., & Hester, P.P. (1994). Generalized effects of milieu teaching. *Journal of Speech Hearing Research, 37,* 1320–1340.

Koegel, R.L., & Koegel, L.K. (2006). *Pivotal response treatments for autism: Communication, social, and academic development.* Baltimore: Paul H. Brookes Publishing Co.

Lovaas, O.I. (1987). Behavioral treatment and normal educational and intellectual functioning in young autistic children. *Journal of Consulting and Clinical Psychology, 55,* 3–9.

Millan, C., & Peltier, M.J. (2007). *Cesar's way: The natural, everyday guide to understanding and correcting common dog problems.* New York: Three Rivers Press.

Pretti-Frontczak, K., & Bricker, D. (2004). *An activity-based approach to early intervention* (3rd ed.). Baltimore: Paul H. Brookes Publishing Co.

Prizant, B., Wetherby, A.M., Rubin, M.S., & Laurent, A.C. (2004). *The SCERTS® Model: Enhancing communication and socioemotional abilities of children with autism spectrum disorder.* Baltimore: Paul H. Brookes Publishing Co.

Rayner, K., Foorman, B.R., Perfetti, C.A., Pesetsky, D., & Seidenberg, M.S. (2001). How psychological science informs teaching of reading. *Psychological Science in the Public Interest, 2,* 31–74.

Stahmer, A.C., Schreibman, L., & Cunningham, A.B. (2010). Towards a technology of treatment individualization for young children with autism spectrum disorders. *Brain Research.* September 18, 2010. Advance Online Publication. PMID: 20858466

Stuebing, K.K., Barth, A.E., Cirino, P.T., Francis, D.J., & Fletcher, J.M. (2008). A response to recent reanalyses of the National Reading Panel Report: Effects of systematic phonics instruction are practically significant. *Journal of Educational Psychology, 199,* 123–134.

Thompson, T. (2007). *Dr. Thompson's straight talk on autism.* Baltimore: Paul H. Brookes Publishing Co.

Acknowledgments

Chapters 7–10 were collaborations with Lisa M. Barsness, Clinic Director, and Beth Burggraff, Clinical Supervisor, as well as Patti L. Dropik, Clover A. Anderson, and Amy Bohannan, all Senior Behavior Therapists at the Minnesota Early Autism Project (MEAP) at the time. They all have completed master's degrees and have an average of 15 years of experience in our field. I am most grateful to them for their insights and written contributions and their creativity and dedication to the children we have together served. Thanks, too, to the remarkably competent therapists who, day in and day out, work to improve the lives of children with autism with whom we work.

I would like to express my gratitude to the children and families with whom I have worked and from whom I have learned so much. They are a continual source of inspiration. Special thanks to Terra Hyatt, mother of Jessi; Deanna, mother of Leo; Emily Dalbec, mother of Blake; and Cindy Tupy and Doug Green, parents of Lilly, whose comments about their experience with their children's intensive early behavior therapy are included in Chapters 7–10. Their generosity in sharing their thoughts and feelings is enormously appreciated. Thanks, too, to Dr. Jack Fletcher on his helpful comments on reading research on the Preface.

Finally, I would like to thank Paul H. Brookes Publishing Co. Senior Acquisitions Editor Rebecca Lazo and Editorial Director Heather Shrestha for their continuing support. I am grateful for their confidence in my ability to communicate with Brookes Publishing Co.'s readers. Thanks also to Associate Editor Steve Plocher and Senior Production Editor Leslie Eckard, whose adroit word craft greatly improved the quality of the manuscript.

To the memory of my friend Ted Carr,
who taught us so much about compassionate science
in the service of children with autism

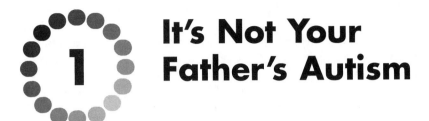

It's Not Your Father's Autism

"You cannot step twice into the same stream."

—Plato, *Cratylus, On the Nature of Things* (1921)

This book addresses the individual differences among children with autism, which require individualizing interventions that match child characteristics. Although some children require highly structured approaches and others need interventions that are embedded in typical daily routines, many children benefit most from *Blended Interventions,* combinations of these approaches. In order to better understand which children make the greatest gains with each of these strategies, we must first understand the sources of variation among children diagnosed with Autism Spectrum Disorders (ASDs). We begin by reviewing autism subtypes and how our understanding of them has changed since the condition was first described.

AUTISM SUBTYPES

Autism is a family of disabilities sharing several common features but differing considerably in other ways, which creates complications for parents and professionals alike. In this chapter, I examine origins of the diagnostic label *autism;* review current diagnostic standards, and introduce the notion that there are subtypes of autism, which has important implications for choice of intervention. The term *autism* has evolved over the last century. First introduced by Kraeplin in 1919 to refer to a symptom of schizophrenia (then known as *dementia praecox*), the diagnostic label of *autism* has been found in the *Diagnostic and Statistical Manual of Mental Disorders* through the *Fourth Edition, Text Revision (DSM-IV-TR;* American Psychiatric Association [APA], 2000), but changes to the terminology are pending in the fifth edition to be published in 2013 (APA, 2010).

This Isn't Your Father's Autism

Parents of children with autism often feel like Dorothy in the movie *The Wizard of Oz* (LeRoy & Fleming, 1939). Dorothy famously said to her pet terrier, "Toto, I've a feeling we're not in Kansas anymore." Parents find themselves in the vortex of a diagnostic maelstrom, and when they land, it is in equally unfamiliar territory. As their child's pediatrician or psychologist discusses their child's diagnostic findings, parents hear a litany of unfamiliar terms, such as *insistence on sameness, joint attention,* and *stereotyped mannerisms.* Autism is a world replete with obscure words and concepts.

When well-meaning professionals deliver the shocking news to parents that their child has an ASD, the parents' minds shut down as the ominous word *autism* reverberates in their heads. During that initial discussion, the remainder of what professionals subsequently say has about as much impact as the chatter of the Munchkins in the Land of Oz. Parents vainly hope to hear encouraging words from the doctor suggesting that this is just a minor fork in the road of their child's otherwise typical development. Instead, the doctor tells the parents, with an implicit sense of urgency, that they should apply for an early intervention program for their child as soon as possible. There is a note of tension in the doctor's voice as she tries not to add to the parents' distress. Parents sense that the clock is ticking.

"I've seen the truth, and it makes no sense," a father thinks. Parents desperately wish things could be a lot simpler, like in the "good old days." It turns out that, although autism diagnosis was simpler in the old days, it was also often wrong by today's standards. What a condition is called, and what it *actually is,* can make a world of difference.

Autism in the "Good Old Days"

"I don't get it," a frustrated father says. "Does our son have autism or doesn't he?" Several decades ago, the answer parents received from doctors was a lot simpler to understand, but it was often incorrect, at least based on our current understanding. In the past, autism was considered to be a single condition, a form of childhood psychosis. Over the past 30 years it has become clear that autism (or ASD, which is what most people currently mean when they use the term *autism*) is actually *a group of interrelated brain developmental disorders* that share three basic features (socialization challenges, communication challenges, and restricted repetitive behavior), but differ considerably as disorders. So when the exasperated dad asks whether his son has autism, the answer 30 years ago may very likely have been, "No, he doesn't have autism," because in that era, researchers had identified only the most severe forms of *Autistic Disorder,* as these developmental disorders were then called. Today the psychologist's, pediatrician's, or child psychiatrist's reply may be that the child has *a form of autism spectrum disorder,* which might be very different from other types. The child may talk and express interest in other children. He may not strike his head with his fists or bite his hands. But the child may be unable to initiate and sustain a social interaction, and he may line up his toy cars and have tantrums if they are disrupted. He may exhibit little eye contact and ignore other children's attempts to play with him. The child's doctor explains that he has a milder form of an ASD. Which subtype of ASD the child has will play an important role in deciding what kind of treatment is likely to have the greatest impact. Parents soon discover that a simple black-and-white answer isn't in the cards.

From the 1960s until around 1980, the public's impression of autism was created largely by motion pictures or made-for-television dramas depicting a typical child trapped inside an impervious psychological shell, waiting to be freed. Autism was popularly portrayed as a severe withdrawal from reality, during which the nonverbal child rocked and hand-flapped, twirled in circles, often struck his or her own head, screamed and bit, and did not tolerate being touched. Youngsters diagnosed with autism were described as "psychotic children," not only in fictional depictions but in medical publications, as well. Cinematic images ranged from Francois Truffaut's *L'Enfant Sauvage* (*The Wild Child*; Berbert & Truffaut, 1970) to *Change of Habit* (Connelly & Graham, 1969), in which Elvis Presley played a doctor to whom a girl with autism was brought for treatment. The girl resisted being held, did not respond when spoken to, and incessantly rocked. A kindly and sensitive Elvis treated the girl with understanding and warmth, and she miraculously began to "break out of her autism." That was a common plot line in early depictions of autism treatment: A compassionate psychotherapist or social worker, by some unspecified means, coaxed the child out of her shell back into normalcy. As appealing as that image may be, experience has taught us that this is not the best way to help a child overcome his or her autism symptoms.

Truffaut's film presented the story of Dr. Jean Itard's encounter with a 12-year-old feral boy with autism in 1798 and Itard's attempts to cure the boy, whom he named Victor. The film was based on Itard's book *The Wild Boy of Aveyron* (1962), and though the film was a dramatization, it was a reasonably accurate rendering of Itard's clinical description. Unlike the "magical mystery cures" so often portrayed in many fictional motion pictures, Truffaut's film accurately portrayed Victor as making great strides under Itard's care, but continuing to have a significant disability even after the prescient doctor had worked with him for several years.

The reality of those days was very different from the movie version for children with autism. Only children with symptoms we now associate with severe ASDs were diagnosed with autism, and they were often first brought to professional attention about the time the child entered kindergarten or first grade. Generally, early intervention did not exist. Although some affluent families could afford to take their sons or daughters with autism to child psychoanalysts or costly residential retreats, the vast majority of children with autism received no special intervention at all. I don't recall ever hearing of a child with autism who was extricated from his or her disability via psychoanalytic play therapy. On school entry, most children with autism, if they were nonverbal or repeatedly vocalized or said words that made no sense, were placed in classrooms for students with severe intellectual disabilities, such as Down syndrome, or a brain injury, such as that caused by bacterial meningitis. If they were higher functioning and verbal, they were often placed in classrooms for children who were severely emotionally disturbed, some of whom were violent. Though their teachers likely tried valiantly to teach their students basic functional skills, the results were usually discouraging for the child, his or her parents, and teachers.

In 1967, autism was classified as a type of schizophrenia, and what few treatments were available were based on the assumption that autism was closely related to that major psychotic disorder. It isn't. That was an unfortunate mistake that misled many parents, doctors, therapists, and teachers to adopt treatments usually used for severely psychotic adults. The diagnostic picture began to change in 1980 when, for the first time, the *Diagnostic and Statistical Manual of Mental Disorders, Third Edition* (DSM-III; APA, 1980) cleaved autism from schizophrenia, categorizing the condition as a developmental disorder. It was no longer considered a psychotic disorder. Autism continued to be thought of as a single condition until 1994, when the *Diagnostic and Statistical Manual of Mental Disorders, Fourth Edition* (DSM-IV; APA, 1994) introduced Asperger's Disorder as a separate condition, and subsequently added Pervasive Developmental Disorder-Not Otherwise Specified (PDD-NOS; called *Atypical Autism* outside the United States) to the list of Autism Spectrum Disorders. Finally it was recognized that earlier caricatures of autism as a form of severe withdrawal from reality, accompanied by extremely bizarre behavior, lack of speech, and violent behavior, were highly inaccurate for a large portion of children on the autism spectrum. Although all children with ASDs have social and language deficits and some ritualistic behavior, the motion picture versions of the past were clearly very misleading.

Who Cares What You Call It; Just Fix My Kid!

We have become an exceedingly impatient culture. As an example, if an Internet web site's home page requires more than a few seconds to load, today's average web surfer moves on to another web site. We have come to expect simple, instant responses to our questions without being bothered with what we view to be ancillary information: "Don't bother me with all the technical details," people say. When the television meteorologist points to lines on the map and says, "A low-pressure zone is moving in from the southwest containing moisture from the Gulf, colliding with a high-pressure Alberta clipper," our eyes glaze over and we quickly flip the channel. "Just tell me whether it's going to rain, and how much," we think.

Parents of children with ASDs often view diagnostic information with similar impatience. It is understandable that parents want simple "yes-or-no" answers. Often, the language of science flummoxes them: "I don't want to hear all of that medical and psychological mumbo jumbo; just tell me what's wrong with him and what to do about it," an overwhelmed mother may think. The problem is that the best course of intervention for a child with an ASD often very much depends on that scientific "mumbo jumbo," the technical distinctions among a child's symptoms, and autism subtypes. We are approaching an era in autism intervention that some other advanced areas of medicine have already reached. For instance, in cancer treatment, today's specialists need to know a great deal about the type of cancer the individual has, often including its genetic code, how it spreads in the body, the size of the lesion, and so forth, before deciding on a course of treatment. In autism services, we are clearly heading in a similar direction. The pathway from initial diagnosis to implementing an effective intervention for a child with autism is often circuitous, with fits and starts, and can be greatly aided by developing a "road map." The process is seldom linear; you can't just draw a straight line from where you are now to where you would like to be.

For the purposes of this book, I will cut through as much technical jargon as possible to get to the core information that practitioners and parents need to understand their child's condition and more rationally weigh intervention options. But be forewarned: It isn't possible to avoid all scientific language. The fundamental question is, "What type of ASD does this child have?" Once we better understand a child's autism profile, we need to know whether there are other factors that should be considered in choosing an intervention. The answers to these questions lead the way to achieving a better understanding of intervention options—and their likely outcomes.

Current Autism Diagnosis

Medical diagnosis refers to "the process of determining the nature of a disease, etc.; the identification of a disease from the patient's symptoms; a formal statement of this" (Brown, 1993, p. 660), and generally includes *differential diagnosis,* in other words, the process of weighing how likely it is a person has one disease versus other diseases with similar symptoms that could account for the person's condition. For the purposes of ASD interventions, medical diagnosis is not the same as *educational identification.* Schools conduct testing that is similar to medical diagnostic testing to determine whether a child is likely to profit from educational services for an ASD. Educational systems are unlikely to conduct differential diagnostic evaluations, because they may involve ruling out other medical conditions such as epilepsy as a cause of the child's symptoms, and diagnosing such medical conditions is usually outside the competence of school personnel. If a child scores within a specified range on diagnostic tests and classroom observations seem consistent with autism, the child is qualified for autism educational services.

Medical diagnostic information is used for several purposes. A diagnosis makes it possible to better understand the course of the condition, its prognosis, and how good the outcome is likely to be. That is important for helping families understand what to expect and to plan. Differential diagnosis permits the clinician to determine the most appropriate interventions for the condition (e.g., for autism versus selective mutism) and their likely outcomes. Diagnostic information is also used by federal and state agencies and private insurance companies to determine whether, and to what degree, reimbursement will be provided for various treatments for a given disease or disorder. There are also public health and research implications of accurate diagnosis. If we want to determine whether a given form of therapy is beneficial to children with autism, it is essential that the diagnostic criteria used for including participants in the study be clearly specified. If not, the study sample might inadvertently include a mixture of children with a variety of conditions (e.g., attention-deficit/hyperactivity disorder [ADHD], speech-language disorders, obsessive-compulsive disorder), making the results uninterpretable. Pediatricians, child psychiatrists, pediatric neurologists, and licensed psychologists usually make formal medical diagnoses of ASDs.

Medical diagnostic assessments for various disorders or disabilities differ greatly depending on the condition being evaluated. Generally, a symptom or group of symptoms leads parents of a child affected by autism to seek assistance from a physician. For example, Brandon, a 3-year-old child, isn't talking, shows little interest in people, and has frequent tantrums. There is no single medical test that will determine whether Brandon has autism. With some disorders, a single diagnostic test, such as a magnetic resonance imaging (MRI) scan of the person's brain, together with an evaluation of his or her symptoms, may be sufficient to arrive at a tentative diagnosis (e.g., a 65-year-old man has had a stroke). In many other instances, the diagnostic test results are only interpretable with knowledge of the person's history and, possibly, additional tests.

There are no brain scans, electroencephalograms, blood tests, or other laboratory tests for ASDs. Diagnosis is made based on the child's history, testing completed by a mental health professional based on observing the child, and completion of rating scales by the child's parents and teachers that cover major domains of the child's history and development. Diagnosis can be facilitated by information from the family history, because some forms of autism run in families. Tests of speech-language development and intellectual development, and at times other neuropsychological tests, may assist with differential diagnosis to rule out other developmental problems. Occasionally, differential diagnosis may also require assessment with a brain wave test to rule out an epileptic disorder, or with an MRI scan to make certain the child does not have other brain conditions that could resemble some features of ASDs.

Diagnostic Systems

When parents receive a written diagnostic report from their child's doctor or psychologist, the summary section often reads something like this: "Kevin's history and current symptoms are consistent with a diagnosis of Autistic Disorder (299.0)." This sentence contains two pieces of information about Kevin's diagnosis: 1) The diagnostic label of Autistic Disorder used by the APA in the *DSM-IV-TR*, and 2) the corresponding numerical code (299.0) used by the World Health Organization's *International Statistical Classification of Diseases and Related Health Problems, 10th Revision (ICD-10;* 1992), which is also used in the United States for administrative purposes such as insurance claims.

Autism Clinical Syndromes

Three clinical ASDs are described in the *DSM-IV-TR* and *ICD-10*, the most current versions as of this writing: Autistic Disorder, PDD-NOS (or Atypical Autism), and Asperger's Disorder. As noted earlier, the latter two categories may be eliminated in the *DSM-V* when it is published in 2013. All three clinical conditions involve problems in developing age-appropriate communication and social skills, but to varying degrees. The third category of symptoms refers to the tendency to engage in repetitive movements or rigid routine activities that serve no practical function, such as rocking, flicking fingers before one's eyes, or repeatedly flipping light switches. The following case examples illustrate typical patterns of core symptoms of individuals receiving diagnoses within the three major ASDs, as they would be revealed by standardized diagnostic assessment during a typical clinical evaluation.

• • • • • • • • • •

AUTISTIC DISORDER

Madison, who is 3 years, 10 months old, was assessed to determine her eligibility for intensive early behavior intervention services. Madison's previous assessment by her public school's Early Childhood Special Education program revealed that her intellectual developmental score was at the first percentile (i.e., nearly all children her age scored higher than Madison) and her language scores were at 8 and 11 months, respectively, well below her chronological age. An independent licensed psychologist conducted an Autism Diagnostic Observation Schedule (ADOS) assessment (Lord, Rutter, DiLavore, & Risi, 1999; considered the diagnostic "gold standard") and found that Madison's score indicated she would qualify for an Autistic Disorder diagnosis if the remaining findings were consistent with this conclusion. In each of the following sections, phrases in italics are signs or symptoms that, if endorsed based on the observation and interview, are consistent with an autism spectrum diagnosis.

Communication Domain

Madison has a *significant language/speech delay and has limited ability to communicate her needs and wants.* She occasionally says a few words, such as "more," "no," "baby," and "bye-bye." She *makes no attempt to initiate a conversation with her parents or her brother.* She makes occasional *repetitive speech* sounds or short phrases, but they *do not seem to serve a communicative function;* they seem to be a form of repetitive self-stimulation. She exhibits *no make-believe play.* She *does not participate in back-and-forth conversation, and she does not use or respond to gestures.*

Social Domain

Madison *occasionally exhibits brief eye-to-eye gaze* with her parents but no one else. She *does not respond appropriately to parent gestures* (e.g., beckoning to "come here"). She *shows little interest in other children* and doesn't initiate interactions with them. She *occasionally holds up items she is playing with to her parents and makes a simultaneous vocalization* that they are unable to understand. She exhibits *no social reciprocity,* such as taking turns. She *does not react to other's emotions.* She carries a doll with her, but *does not use it for imaginative play.* Madison exhibits aggression toward children at school, her younger brother Andy, and occasionally even unfamiliar children. Her parents report that these outbursts occur more often when she is frustrated.

Repetitive Behavior and Fixed Routines

Madison exhibits *repetitive or perseverative behavior* that is disturbing to her family, potentially dangerous, and stigmatizing. She frequently *places inappropriate objects in her mouth, and holds pieces of cloth, threads, or paper in both hands and walks around shaking them*, occasionally waving them. She refuses to give up the items she is holding without a tantrum. She also dumps crayons or other small items out of a bin or box, puts them back in the bin, and then dumps them again, repeatedly. Her parents report that she periodically has severe "meltdowns" that last for up to 45 minutes. Although some of these outbursts seem to be in response to frustration, at other times parents are unable to identify anything that triggered them. Madison *appears to be frightened of loud sounds,* running and hiding or seeking reassurance when they occur.

● ● ● ● ● ● ● ● ● ●

PERVASIVE DEVELOPMENTAL DISORDER-NOT OTHERWISE SPECIFIED

Carter is 4 years, 9 months old and lives with his mother, father, brother (6 years old), and sister (2 years old). His parents noticed that something was different about his development at about 18 months of age when he *showed no interest in other children and wasn't talking yet*. His parents brought him for this evaluation so that they could determine what services he might need. Intellectual assessment indicates that Carter functions in the low average range. His language test scores place him somewhat lower, though his understanding of what people say to him is superior to his ability to engage in meaningful spoken communication. The Vineland Adaptive Behavior Scales (VABS; Sparrow, Cicchetti, & Balla, 2005) indicate that all of his skills are average or low average except communication, which is lower. The Conners Scale for Attention Deficit Hyperactivity Disorder (Conners, 2008) was administered, and Carter scored in the clinically significant range for the Combined Type of ADHD.

Social Domain

At the evaluation, Carter was very *socially outgoing* and almost immediately responded to overtures from the examiner. He enjoyed blowing bubbles and trying to catch them. He *exhibited relatively complex imaginative play*. He exhibited *limited eye contact*. He *showed toys to his mother and to the examiner*. He rapidly switched his attention from one toy to another, often tossing the first one and immediately picking up a second. He climbed on top of a table and tipped over a chair and pushed it around the room as if it were a vehicle. His mother reported that he interacts with his brother in rough-and-tumble play but seldom with other children. His mother reported that Carter and his brother occasionally take turns, but usually not with other children or adults. His mother said that he periodically hits, scratches, or pinches his brother or sister, usually over access to toys. He becomes very impatient and grabs toys from them and shoves or hits them. He does not seem to notice when his sister is crying. He shows no reaction to other people's facial expressions.

Communication Domain

Almost immediately on entering the assessment room, Carter *began talking with the examiner* and playing with various toys. He *answered questions with single words or short phrases*. He *used some gestures, such as pointing,* to supplement his spoken communication attempts. He didn't participate in multipart conversational exchanges. His *spoken language is delayed,* with articulation problems for which he is receiving speech therapy. *No stereotyped or repetitive use of language or echolalia was observed.*

Repetitive Behavior and Fixed Routines

His mother reported that Carter *has few fixed routines* and seldom becomes upset if there is a change in routine. He will not eat meat, although otherwise he is a good eater. *No motor mannerisms, such as flapping, twirling, or rocking* were observed, though his mother reports that at 2 years of age he frequently twirled in a circle and looked up at overhead lamps. That no longer occurs. His mother reports that his main problem is his impulsiveness and high activity level, combined with his *lack of social understanding,* which creates problems with other children.

● ● ● ● ● ● ● ● ● ●

ASPERGER SYNDROME

Rachel, who is 5 years, 6 months old was evaluated for possible ASD. A preschool and primary school intellectual assessment test was administered, yielding a full-scale IQ score of 117—in the high average range. On another developmental test, Rachel's *communication and cognitive abilities were well above average.* Rachel's Combined Adaptive Behavior score was average, while her personal social and motor scores were quite low. The ADOS was completed, and Rachel's score was in the Autism Spectrum range, but below the Autistic Disorder range.

Social Skills Domain

At the evaluation, Rachel had no difficulty separating from her mother and joining a therapist on the floor of the assessment room to play with toys. She *exhibited occasional eye contact* with a therapist and once, fleetingly, with the examiner. She *readily initiated interactions with the therapist* but did not seem to wait for the therapist's responses before continuing with her play, seemingly oblivious to what the therapist had said. She *did not use gestures or seem to respond to others' gestures.* Her mother reported that Rachel *has interest in peers but does not know how to initiate or maintain social interactive play.* Her mother says Rachel occasionally *shows her an object that interests her.* She *became agitated and began crying when the therapist attempted to change the theme of her ongoing play.* After about a half hour, she asked her mother whether it was time to leave. Her mother says she *does not react appropriately to others' emotions.* She becomes upset when her brother cries, but only because she dislikes the sound of crying. If he continues crying, at times she hits him. Although she enjoys affection from her parents, she *shows no empathy.* She *has no tolerance for turn taking and has emotional outbursts when she loses at games.*

Communication Domain

Rachel began to use speech functionally when she was 14 months old. Then her speech seemed to "explode." She *seemed to understand most things adults said to her, with a vocabulary well beyond her age.* Her *spontaneous expressive communication was often tangential and involved unusual "made-up" words.* At the evaluation, practitioners noted that she appeared to enjoy creating rhyming words, such as "Hickory dickory duck, the mouse ran up the pluck." Her rhyming speech has a musical quality. She asked a few appropriate questions and responded more or less appropriately within her play context. She *exhibited make-believe play,* but her mother reports that her imaginative play is limited to a couple of topics and she *becomes very frustrated if anyone tries to change the topic.* She often *narrated or commented on her play* or other actions during the clinical observation, which involved dolls or animals riding on a merry-go-round. Although this is common for children her age who are typically developing, it is unusual for most young children on the autism spectrum. During these narrations, she used *unusual words for a child her age,* such as "remarkable," "conquer," and "acceptable."

Repetitive Behavior and Fixed Routines

Rachel *did not engage in obvious motor stereotypic behavior, such as flapping, twirling, or finger flicking.* She *occasionally engaged in "edging,"* looking out of the corner of her eye along elongated lines, which is a form of visual self-stimulation. Her mother reports she *has several fixed routines* (e.g., getting ready for bed) that must be followed precisely or she has a meltdown. Occasionally *during meltdowns she scratches her face and body with her fingernails.*

Rachel's parents are told her precocious language skills, combined with significant social skill limitations and excessive need for control over daily routines and associated emotional outbursts, are consistent with an Asperger disorder diagnosis. While some children with Asperger disorder have unusually high intelligence, most have intellectual functioning within the average to high average range like Rachel.

● ● ● ● ● ● ● ● ●

Commentary

Although these diagnostic categories of ASDs are important, they alone cannot serve as the basis for an intervention plan. The formal diagnosis is only a first step. Within each of these clinical categories are wide variations of expression, from a child exhibiting no speech who may be on the severe end of the autism spectrum, to a child in middle school with High-Functioning Autistic Disorder speaking in complete sentences. Moreover, the expression of adaptive abilities as well as deficits depends in part on associated developmental challenges such as ADHD, serious anxiety problems, or speech-language disorder. Sorting out the sources of differences is the major thrust of this part of the book.

Types of Autism Based on Physical Features

Dr. Judith Miles is Professor of Pediatrics at the University of Missouri Medical School in Columbia. She has devoted much of her career to trying to better understand children's genetic disorders. Some time ago, Dr. Miles and I were part of a panel at a conference on children's disabilities. During a break in the proceedings, she told me about interesting findings that were emerging in her autism clinic, making notations of her findings on a coffee-stained paper napkin as she did so. I was stunned by what she told me.

Children seen in Miles's clinic for autism evaluation received a multidisciplinary evaluation, from brain scans to blood workups to language and psychological testing. Miles began noticing that children diagnosed with autism fell into two discrete and nearly nonoverlapping groups based on their physical features. Those two groups had very divergent characteristics. Around two-thirds of the children physically resembled other members of their families. These children tended to have milder language and social disabilities, and had higher intelligence test scores than those in the other group. They had fewer brain differences when tested with brain scan or brain wave tests. They generally responded better to behavioral therapies or educational interventions. Her most striking finding was that *children in this group were much more likely to have brothers or sisters or other relatives with autism than children in the second group.*

The remaining one third of children evaluated at Miles's clinic had either smaller head size or somewhat unusual physical features that were *not* similar to others in their families, like unusually placed ears, oddly spaced teeth, wider spaces between eyebrows, or lack of creases in the palm of their hands. These are called *dysmorphic features*. Those children generally had more severe autism symptoms, were more likely to have brain differences when scanned with an MRI or brain wave test, and were more likely to have epilepsy. Miles referred to the second group of children as having *Complex Autism*. It was less likely that autism ran in their families as compared with the first group, which Dr. Miles referred to as having *Essential Autism*. The male-to-female ratio in the Complex Autism group was 3.2 to 1 instead of 6.5 to 1 for the Essential Autism group. Autism symptoms also occur among individuals with other developmental disabilities, such as fragile X syndrome, fetal alcohol syndrome, and Down syndrome; this dual diagnosis is called *Syndromic Autism*. Dr. Miles found that all cases of children with Syndromic Autism fell within the Complex Autism group.

Dr. Miles's findings are important for two reasons. First, they suggest autism symptoms can be caused in at least two very different ways, either by apparent gene inheritance or error, or by something that causes the cells of a developing fetus to begin dividing abnormally while in the womb (e.g., exposure to certain drugs or alcohol, infectious diseases, or maternal diabetes or other hormone problems). Many unusual physical features can also be caused by genetic errors, but when that occurs, various parts of the body are usually affected, producing cleft palate, heart defects, or hand or limb abnormalities rather than mainly differences in brain development.

As we will see shortly, children who fall into the Essential Autism group appear to have failed to develop normal connections in critical brain structures, which can be at least in part remediated by early intervention. Damage to some of the same brain areas associated with Complex Autism appears to be less amenable to improvement through social intervention. That suggests a different type of developmental error has occurred, even though it produces some of the same symptoms.

Relation to Early Intervention Outcome

In 2005, the same year Miles and her colleagues published their first report (Miles et al., 2005), Dr. Glen Sallows and Tamylnn Graupner, directors of the Wisconsin Early Autism Project in Madison, published results of another important study. Sallows and Graupner reported outcomes for 24 children with autism who had received 4 years of intensive early behavioral intervention, including cognitive, language, adaptive, social, and academic measures. They found that 48% of the children showed rapid learning, achieved post-intervention scores in the average range compared with their peers who were typically developing, and at age 7 were succeeding in regular education classrooms. The rest of the children were moderate or slow learners who showed many fewer gains with respect to core autism symptoms and intellectual functioning (Sallows & Graupner, 2005). Figure 1.1 shows the progress of children in the two groups. The rapid-learning children achieved remarkable gains within 1–2 years, while the second group showed much less progress with the same intervention over 4 years. Sallows and

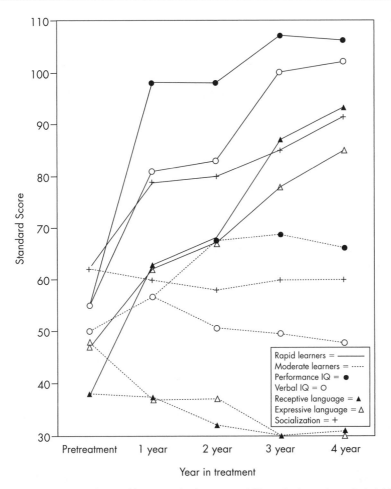

Figure 1.1. Measures of IQ and language development in children who learned rapidly (solid lines) and who learned more slowly (dashed lines) in an intensive early behavioral intervention study. Rapid learners exhibited marked increases in language and intellectual functioning within 1–2 years, although those who learned more slowly showed limited improvement with the same intensity and duration of intervention. (From Sallows, G.O., & Graupner, T.D. [2005]. Intensive behavioral treatment for children with autism: Four-year outcome and predictors. *American Journal of Mental Retardation, 110*[6], 427; reprinted by permission.)

Graupner were not aware of Judith Miles's work at the time of their study, and as a result had not attempted to measure head size or obtain other medical measures of their participants. However, the outcomes for their two distinctively different groups mirror those of the Miles and colleagues' (2005) Essential and Complex Autism groups, though the percentages of the whole in each group are somewhat different. Sallows and Graupner's findings, like Miles's, suggest that the group of children with Essential Autism exhibit a developmental error in brain connectivity (synapse formation) that can be substantially overcome by intensive social intervention. The second group, those with Complex Autism, have neural dysfunctions that require a more functionally based intervention approach designed to develop communication and daily living skills, but which may have less effect on core autism symptoms.

Choice of intervention is based on the balance of core autism features, intellectual functioning, and attention limitations, which differ among autism subtypes. In Chapter 2, I will discuss autism's multidimensional nature and examine a strategy for evaluating those dimensions for children on the autism spectrum.

SUMMARY

Our understanding of what autism is has changed dramatically since the mid-1980s. It is not a psychotic condition like schizophrenia. It appears there are broad differences in types of autism with apparently different causes. The most common appear to be either inherited genetic causes or mutations—spontaneous genetic errors. A smaller subset of autism seems to be caused by such things as infections, exposure to toxins such as alcohol during pregnancy, or other health conditions such as hormone abnormalities. The three clinical syndromes—Autistic Disorder, PDD-NOS, and Asperger syndrome—describe a continuum of ASDs varying widely in their combination of features, but all show difficulties with communication, social skills, and repetitive nonfunctional routines.

REFERENCES

American Psychiatric Association. (1980). *Diagnostic and statistical manual of mental disorders* (3rd ed.). Washington, DC: Author.

American Psychiatric Association. (1994). *Diagnostic and statistical manual of mental disorders* (4th ed.). Washington, DC: Author.

American Psychiatric Association. (2000). *Diagnostic and statistical manual of mental disorders* (4th ed., text revision). Washington, DC: Author.

American Psychiatric Association. (2010). DSM-V: The future of psychiatric diagnosis. *DSM-5 Development.* Retrieved March 6, 2010, from http://www.psych.org/dsmv.aspx

Berbert, M. (Producer), & Truffaut, F. (Director). (1970). *L'Enfant sauvage* (The Wild Child) [Motion picture]. France: Les Films du Carrosse.

Brown, L. (Ed.). (1993). *The new shorter Oxford English dictionary.* New York: Oxford University Press.

Connelly, J. (Producer), & Graham, W.A. (Director). (1969). *Change of habit* [Motion picture]. United States: MCA Universal Pictures.

Conners, C.K. (2008). *Conners–Third Edition (Conners-3).* Toronto, ON: Multi-Health Systems Inc.

Itard, J.M.G. (1962). *The wild boy of Aveyron.* (G.M. Humphrey, Trans.). New York: Appleton-Century-Crofts.

Kraeplin, E. (1919). *Dementia praecox and paraphrenia.* Edinburgh, Scotland: Livingston.

LeRoy, M. (Producer), & Fleming, V. (Director). (1939). *The wizard of Oz* [Motion picture]. United States: Metro-Goldwyn-Mayer.

Lord, C., Rutter, M., DiLavore, P.C., & Risi, S. (1999). *Autism Diagnostic Observation Schedule–WPS Edition.* Los Angeles: Western Psychological Services.

Miles, J.H., Takahashi, T.N., Bagby, S., Sahota, P.K., Vaslow, D.F., Wang, C.H., et al. (2005). Essential versus complex autism: Definition of fundamental prognostic subtypes. *American Journal of Medical Genetics, 135A,* 171–180.

Plato (1921). Cratylus. In *Plato in Twelve Volumes, Vol. 12.* Retrieved Feb. 14, 2010, from http://old.perseus.tufts.edu/cgi-bin/ptext?doc=Perseus%3Atext%3A1999.01.0172

Sallows, G.O., & Graupner, T.D. (2005). Intensive behavioral treatment for children with autism: Four-year outcome and predictors. *American Journal of Mental Retardation, 110*(6), 417–438.

Sparrow, S., Cicchetti, D., & Balla, D. (2005). *Vineland Adaptive Behavior Scales* (2nd ed.). Circle Pines, MN: American Guidance Service.

World Health Organization. (1992). *The ICD-10 classification of mental and behavioural disorders: Clinical descriptions and diagnostic guidelines.* Geneva: Author.

2 Autism Profiles and Blended Intervention

"What is food to one, to others bitter poison."

—Titus Lucretius Carus, *On the Nature of Things* (99–55 b.c.)

We all know there is more to a person than a label such as *Midwesterner, psychologist,* or *watercolor painting enthusiast.* Although such a label may tell us interesting facts about the person, there is a great deal missing (e.g., honesty, generosity, compassion, work ethic, intellectual curiosity) that may tell other, perhaps more important things about a person. Knowing that a child has been given a label, *autistic,* provides more specific information, but other important information is missing that is necessary to begin to plan the most effective intervention for that child. This chapter attempts to put some flesh on the bones of ASD labels. It will consider how best to create a profile of a child with autism by taking into account the whole child, not just the label of ASD, and how to provide interventions based upon that profile. Finally, this chapter will discuss Blended Interventions—using different methods of intervention to address the needs of a particular child.

JEAN ITARD AND LEO KANNER

On January 8, 1800, farmers near the town of Saint-Sernin-sur-Rance, France, brought a struggling and terrified 12-year-old youth, found naked, to a young doctor, Jean Itard. The boy had been seen stealing vegetables and fruit from townspeople and had been captured twice before, but each time he had escaped. On this occasion the youth was turned over to Itard, who specialized in treating deaf children. Itard very quickly recognized that this boy was not like other "mentally disabled" children he had seen. Despite his nakedness, lack of speech, scars on his body, and animal-like eating habits, the feral youth was quite capable in some respects (Itard, 1962). But he exhibited three striking differences from typical children and those with intellectual disabilities, differences that we recognize to this day as the core features of autism: lack of social awareness, communication deficits (or absence of communication), and repetitive behavior and fixed routines.

These core autism features were described in greater detail by Leo Kanner (1943) in his seminal article that first described the clinical syndrome *Early Infantile Autism* in the medical literature. For many years it was believed that the severity of the three features varied together; in other words, if a child's communication deficit was severe, then his or her social skills would be more limited, and it was likely the child would display more intense repetitive compulsive behavior. This reasoning was based largely on the premise that autism was a single condition with a single cause, which we now know is incorrect.

AUTISM VARIABILITY

In selecting the most appropriate intervention for a child, we must take into consideration variability in autism expression. Autism has multiple causes, some inherited, others the result of unpredictable genetic errors called *mutations,* and still others resulting from more global damage to the developing brain, such as that caused by maternal diabetes, hormonal abnormalities, infections, or alcohol or toxin exposure (Gardener, Spiegelman, & Buka, 2009). Despite variability in brain functioning of children with ASDs, numerous studies have shown that several specific brain areas frequently operate atypically. Some of these brain functions can be severely compromised, while others are largely spared. The result is an uneven and difficult-to-predict set of ASD profiles. Dysfunction in various combinations of brain structures can lead to complex profiles of characteristics, which, in turn, have implications for intervention strategy (Thompson, 2007).

AUTISM PROFILES

A *profile* is a pattern of personal characteristics along several dimensions that reliably distinguishes one person from another in important ways and allows us to make predictions about these individuals' future behavior. It is not the same as a *diagnosis,* although profiles are related to diagnoses. Profiles can help identify the combination of characteristics or traits that predict who will be a great long-distance runner, a skillful auto technician, or a child who will learn most effectively through discovery-based preschool instruction. Profiles may also help predict which types of service are most appropriate for a child with autism.

Profiles and Predicting Response to Intervention

Within the field of autism services, having access to a valid profile may enable us to make predictions about a child's behavior under various circumstances, such as which situations will promote new learning and behavior change and which may have a detrimental effect. Constructing profiles depends on knowing the major relevant dimensions along which people of a given type vary, such as teachers, athletes, or children with ASDs. If we created a list of hundreds of phrases that could be used to describe people, such as *hard working, enjoys vegetables,* or *dislikes outdoor sports,* many of those descriptors would not reliably distinguish among people of a given category in a predictive way. Other phrases may critically differentiate among people along important dimensions for a given purpose, such as when considering what type of intervention to provide a child with an ASD. I am concerned here with making predictions about the kinds of teaching or therapy methods that will be most effective for promoting new skills and reducing behavior challenges among children with ASDs and which interventions are likely to be ineffective or perhaps counterproductive.

Creating an *autism intervention profile* begins with identifying core dimensions along which people with an ASD vary, and then examining a child's other characteristics that may moderate the way those dimensions affect their functioning. The core autism dimensions are

· Social skills
· Communication skills
· Tendency to engage in nonfunctional repetitive behavior or to have fixed inflexible interests

Factors that moderate the expression of autism symptoms include

· Intellectual ability and language
· Attention deficit and hyperactivity traits
· Anxiety challenges

A child with autism has many of the same characteristics as any other child.

• • • • • • • • • •

Marina, who will be 4 years old next summer, is diagnosed with PDD-NOS. She has favorite foods like other typically developing children her age—chicken fingers, plain hot dogs, and macaroni and cheese. She refuses to eat many other foods, but so do many other children her age who are typically developing. She fights with her brother over who gets to play with their Fisher Price Little People toys. She is afraid of fire engine sirens and the sound of thunder, which make her cover her ears with her hands, but she is more fearful of those sounds than her typical peers. She likes *Teletubbies* and *SpongeBob SquarePants* television shows, but runs out of the room when the *Transformers* cartoon appears on the screen. And like many other children her age, she often resists going to bed at bedtime.

Marina also has some differences. She has far fewer social interests and skills than other children her age. She lacks understanding of communication, has deficits in language skills compared with her same-age peers, and doesn't seem to fully understand the purpose of spoken communication. She also seems driven to engage in repetitive, nonfunctional routines, such as flapping her hands, spinning in circles, repeatedly opening and closing doors, flipping light switches on and off, and lining up objects (e.g., toy vehicles) and peering at parts of them with great intensity. If those repetitive behavior patterns are interrupted, she often cries and screams and may strike out against the person who disrupted her preferred routine.

• • • • • • • • • •

Autism Dimensions Pyramid

Figure 2.1 shows a pyramid that represents the combination of the three main dimensions of ASDs. Each of the three lines running from the bottom of the pyramid to the top represents one of those three dimensions—socialization, communication, and repetitive behavior. Imagine a dot on each line that you can slide up and down like a bead on a string. The greater the communication or social deficits, the higher on those lines the dots rest. The pointed top of the pyramid represents the most severe symptoms, and the wide triangular bottom represents neurotypical functioning. The dashed-line triangle cutting through the pyramid represents the balance of a child's three primary autism characteristics. The larger the triangle (dashed line) transecting the pyramid, the more neurotypical the child.

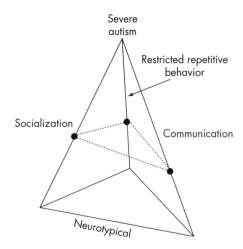

Figure 2.1. A pyramid representing the combination of the three main dimensions of ASDs: socialization, communication, and repetitive behavior. The pointed top of the pyramid represents the most severe symptoms, and the wide triangular bottom represents neurotypical functioning. The balance of a child's three primary autism characteristics is represented by the dashed-line triangle cutting through the pyramid. The larger the triangle (dashed line) transecting the pyramid, the more neurotypical the child.

● ● ● ● ● ● ● ● ●

Jasmine, a 2-year, 10-month-old girl diagnosed with an ASD, has little spoken language, doesn't use gestures, and seldom responds when spoken to. But Jasmine is socially curious, gives her brother a hug when he is crying, and attempts to play with other children, though she doesn't know how to do so. Her socialization dimension score (and corresponding dot) would be between the middle and the bottom of the pyramid—closer to the neurotypical range—but her communication dimension score would be closer to the top—closer to the severe range. She has some compulsive routines, such as flipping light switches, but few tantrums when they are interrupted, so her repetitive behavior dimension score (and its corresponding dot) is midway between the bottom and top. We draw three dashed lines connecting Jasmine's dots. The result is the dashed-line triangle transecting the pyramid that represents Jasmine's autism profile.

● ● ● ● ● ● ● ● ●

A child with autism is a multidimensional individual, and simply saying that the child has autism doesn't begin to help us understand the child or his or her needs. The balance of those three features, and their proximity to the top or bottom of the autism dimensions pyramid, is the starting point in deciding which intervention approach to use.

INTELLECTUAL ABILITY AND LANGUAGE SKILLS

A child's balance of core autism symptoms is an important part of deciding which intervention approach to take, but it is not the whole story. A child's intellectual ability is correlated with response to early intervention methods. Scores on standardized language tests are positively correlated with intellectual ability. For example, Alex's language test score is well below the midpoint of the average range. If Alex also has a socialization score in the mid-range or higher, he may profit from more naturalistic (incidental) Early Intensive Behavioral Intervention (EIBI). But we have to consider additional factors before reaching that conclusion. Such children are more likely to process information more rapidly and generalize to similar, but not identical, situations that are common in naturalistic interventions. As important as intellectual ability and language skills are, another set of factors also needs to be taken into consideration: issues of attention.

ATTENTION DEFICIT AND HYPERACTIVITY SYMPTOMS

Although all children with autism have some difficulties focusing their attention, some have much more significant ADHD symptoms. Despite a child's relatively strong language and social skills, he or she may learn more slowly than expected if he or she also has significant ADHD symptoms, such as attention difficulties, hyperactivity, and impulsiveness, all of which can alter our choice of early intervention approach.

Because language skills are usually limited in autism, some ADHD characteristics that depend on language are important primarily among higher functioning children with functional language skills. Take, for example, a child who does not seem to listen when spoken to and does not follow through on instructions, often talks excessively, often interrupts others and may blurt out answers before a question has been completed, or has difficulty waiting his or her turn. These language-dependent ADHD symptoms are seldom seen among children with greater language limitations.

Among children with more significant language and social limitations, other indicators of ADHD symptoms may be of concern. For example, a child may often fail to pay attention to tasks, may have difficulty sustaining attention when playing a game, may avoid or leave activities that require sustained attention, or may simply be easily distracted. Such a child often fidgets and runs around the room when he or she has been asked to remain seated, climbs on or under furniture, moves constantly as if he or she is "on the go," or butts into games or interrupts others.

A child with autism who has more social and language limitations who exhibits a combination of ADHD symptoms like those listed above will probably learn best using a more structured *Discrete Trial Intervention* (DTI) approach. Even among higher functioning children with ADHD symptoms, a *Blended Intervention* (a combination of Discrete Trial and *Incidental Intervention*) approach is likely to be more effective than a purely naturalistic incidental teaching approach. When a new skill is first being introduced, such as using appropriate prepositions (e.g., *in, on, under, beside*), a DTI approach is likely to be effective. Once the child has begun to participate regularly in that learning or therapy task, a more naturalistic intervention, such as embedding preposition use within a theme-based activity, can be gradually introduced.

ANXIETY CHALLENGES

A final major factor in developing an autism intervention profile is the pervasiveness of anxiety problems. Fearfulness is part and parcel of having autism. Different children with autism experience an array of fears. The most common is social anxiety around strangers or groups of people, sometimes even familiar people. Some children with autism are anxious about leaving the safety of their home—a condition called *agoraphobia*. Closely related is a child's fear that he or she will be unable to leave a situation he or she finds alarming, such as a crowded shopping mall or a movie theater. Still others are anxious about anything unfamiliar in their environment. For example, Jenna, 3½ years old, who is diagnosed with Autistic Disorder, violently pushed away a new picture book her therapist brought to her therapy session and descended into inconsolable sobbing. The book contained colorful images of baby animals, a topic that is usually appealing to Jenna, but because the book was unfamiliar, she reacted fearfully. After the new animal babies book was left in Jenna's bedroom for a week, she became desensitized to it and began to be interested in looking at the pictures. Jenna's reaction reminds me of the joke, "Just when I was getting used to yesterday, along came today" (Keillor, 2003, p. 14).

Among the more common and visible anxiety-driven behaviors in autism are obsessive-compulsive routines—specific sequences of behavior patterns that must be carried out in a particular way or the child sobs in anguish. Perfectionism is a type of obsessive-compulsive behavior that is common in very bright, higher functioning children. For example, Brad, a 5-year-old with whom we have been working for nearly 2 years, finds being unable to perform any activity less than perfectly a cause for despair. His senior therapist taught him a choice-making activity that she called "Try or Cry." She practiced numerous scenarios with Brad in which he would have difficulty performing an activity well. Before beginning, Brad selected his preferred reinforcer for trying his best. As soon as he began showing signs of resistance or puckering up, the therapist would say, "What's it going to be Brad, try or cry?" She lavished praise on him for trying his best and made certain he promptly received the promised reinforcer. On the few occasions that he cried, she said, in a matter-of-fact tone of voice, "Next time, you're going to try!" Brad's parents praised him for "being such a big boy." Within several weeks Brad's perfectionism was nearly gone. These obsessive-compulsive behaviors can be dramatic and pervasive, interfering with nearly all aspects of daily activities. They can severely interfere with teaching and therapy activities, which is why they need to be taken into consideration in selecting an intervention approach.

Standardized checklists and rating scales can be used to estimate anxiety problems of children with autism, such as Achenbach's Child Behavior Checklist; (Achenbach, 1991) or the Behavior Assessment System for Children (BASC-2; Reynolds & Kamphaus, 2004), though they are nonspecific with regard to the type of anxiety problem a child is experiencing. The Children's Yale-Brown Obsessive Compulsive Scale (Goodman et al., 1989) has been modified for individuals with pervasive developmental disorders and contains only five compulsion severity items, which may be helpful for youngsters with obsessive-compulsive problems (Scahill et al., 2006).

Children with ASDs and predominant anxiety problems thrive on predictability and structure, often making a naturalistic intervention approach less suitable, at least in the beginning. By definition, incidental teaching and naturalistic therapy approaches are constantly changing in less predictable ways. For children with ASDs, changes in materials, routines, or procedures must be made gradually, and the child must be given choices as much as feasible. Often a child's anxiety problems diminish as they become more comfortable with their teacher or therapist and the typical daily routines. In higher functioning children, providing short periods that are less structured can serve as a good way of testing a child's readiness for introducing incidental teaching therapy.

Parents usually want their child with autism to spend time with peers who are typically developing, such as in a private preschool or an early childhood special education classroom. Those settings can be overwhelming for many children with severe anxiety problems, especially social anxiety difficulties. They are typically noisy, with multiple unpredictable social demands. If making the transition to the classroom is preceded in a stepwise fashion by one-to-one and small-group early behavior therapy activities involving other children, a foundation can then be effectively laid, making school participation appropriate later on.

BLENDED BEHAVIORAL INTERVENTIONS

Differences among children on the autism spectrum discussed in this chapter, and expanded upon in subsequent chapters, form the basis for individualizing autism early intervention strategies. The type and intensity of intervention should be directly related to the type and severity of autism symptoms. There is considerable evidence that Autistic Disorder, Asperger syndrome, and PDD-NOS are, in part, points along a symptom severity continuum (Bolte, Westerwald, Holtmann, Freitag, & Poustka, 2011; Myhr, 1998). As stated in Chapter 1, autism diagnosed in children (usually Autistic Disorder) can be divided into two types: Complex (the most severe form) and Essential, a type of autism that runs in families (Miles et al., 2005). Nonverbal learning disabilities (NVLD) overlap considerably with, and in many respects are indistinguishable from, Asperger syndrome (Cederlund & Gillberg, 2004), a milder variation of Autistic Disorder. Finally, children who are siblings of youngsters diagnosed with autism often have milder symptoms that do not rise to the level of clinical autism spectrum diagnosis, which is called the *Broad Autism Phenotype* (Losh et al., 2009).

The intensity and type of early behavioral intervention ranges from services within a regular education classroom with limited supports (e.g., speech-language pathology services) to 30 or more hours per week of home-based, one-to-one intensive Discrete Trial/applied behavior analysis intervention supplemented by speech-language pathology services. Between those extremes of the intensity continuum are Blended Interventions that involve combinations of Discrete Trial and Incidental Teaching Intervention, which differ both in type and intensity of intervention. Children with Asperger syndrome and milder forms of PDD-NOS often profit from largely naturalistic Incidental Teaching Intervention within typical daily activities at home, preschool, and the community. Deciding what combination of interventions is most appropriate for a given child begins with an analysis of his or her profile of individual differences as outlined above. In Chapter 4, a strategy is presented for weighing these factors as predictors of child outcomes, with some suggested guidelines.

For example, a 3½-year-old boy with PDD-NOS has limited functional spoken language and is socially curious, but lacks social skills. He is inattentive and impulsive, and displays behavioral outbursts when there are unexpected changes in daily routines. He may respond well to a Blended Intervention approach, in which we begin with a series of initial discrete trial tasks conducted at a table or on the floor of the therapy room, such as motor imitation, increased receptive language skills, and object and shape matching. Reinforcers can be access to preferred activities, social interactions with the therapist or teacher (e.g., tickles), or edibles. The goal is to enable the child to learn how to learn (i.e., to grasp the structure of the learning situation). Once he or she is able to focus his attention for longer time periods and to follow adult instructional requests, gradually some of the same tasks will be switched to a more naturalistic format, in which receptive skills are practiced in the context of typical daily activities, such as meal time, playing with a sibling, and so on. Reinforcers will be chosen that are naturally linked to the activities. As the complexity of skills increases, a larger proportion of each daily session will be conducted in an incidental teaching format (i.e., the two interventions will be blended). When new, more difficult skills are introduced, several days or a week of DTI may be used with those new activities, but the remainder will involve incidental teaching methods.

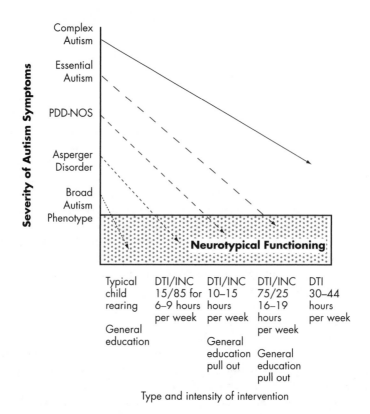

Figure 2.2. Graphic representation of the relationship between severity of autism symptoms, intensity and type of intervention, and likely child outcomes. (Key: DTI = Discrete Trial Intervention, INC = Incidental Intervention)

Figure 2.2 graphically shows the proposed relationship between severity of autism symptoms (vertical axis) and the corresponding intensity and type of intervention and expected child outcomes (horizontal axis). Note that the likelihood of a child outcome falling within the neurotypical range depends on the initial severity of symptoms and the choice of intervention type and intensity.

A child with an ASD who has symptoms associated with one of the diagnostic categories on the vertical axis of this graph may benefit more or less from the type and intensity of intervention indicated, depending on the other moderating factors discussed in this chapter (i.e., ADHD challenges, anxiety problems, more intense compulsive traits, intellectual ability, and language differences). In general, children with more limited language and intellectual functioning generally profit from more emphasis on DTI within a Blended Intervention approach. Children with more severe anxiety problems and repetitive stereotyped behavior also often initially learn more rapidly within a Discrete Trial approach. However, once the child has progressed through the "learning to learn" phase of intervention, greater emphasis on Incidental Intervention approaches is often appropriate. In subsequent chapters, strategies for evaluating these combinations of factors affecting child outcomes are presented in greater detail.

SUMMARY

The diagnostic labels Autistic Disorder, Asperger syndrome, and PDD-NOS are starting points in planning interventions. However, other characteristics also play important roles in developing an autism intervention profile and determining the types of intervention that are likely to be most helpful, whether in isolation or through blending several types of intervention to fit the child. Among the more important are intellectual ability and language skills, ADHD symptoms, and anxiety challenges. The combination and magnitude or severity of these factors provides a framework for beginning to plan an intervention strategy.

REFERENCES

Achenbach, W. (1991). *Child Behavior Checklist, Revised.* Burlington, VT: Achenbach System of Empirically Based Assessment.

Bolte, S., Westerwald, E., Holtmann, M., Freitag, C., & Poustka, F. (2011). Autistic traits and autism spectrum disorders: The clinical validity of two measures presuming a continuum of social communication skills. *Journal of Autism and Developmental Disorders, 41,* 66–72.

Brown, L. (Ed.). (1993). *The New Shorter Oxford English Dictionary.* New York: Oxford University Press.

Carus, T.L. (99–55 b.c.). *On the nature of things, Book IV,* i.637.

Cederlund, M., & Gillberg, C. (2004). One hundred males with Asperger syndrome: A clinical study of background and associated factors. *Developmental Medicine and Child Neurology, 46*(10), 652–660.

Gardener, H., Spiegelman, D., & Buka, S.L. (2009). Prenatal risk factors for autism: Comprehensive meta-analysis. *British Journal of Psychiatry, 195,* 7–14.

Goodman, W.K., Price, L.H., Rasmussen, S.A., Mazure, C., Fleischmann, R.L., Hill, C.L., et al. (1989). The Yale-Brown Obsessive Compulsive Scale. *Archives of General Psychiatry, 46*(11), 1006–1011.

Itard, J. (1962). *The wild boy of Aveyron.* (G.M. Humphrey, Trans.). New York: Appleton Century Crofts.

Kanner, L. (1943). Autistic disturbances of affective contract [Electronic version]. *The Nervous Child, 2,* 217–240.

Keillor, G. (Ed.). (2003). *A Prairie Home Companion pretty good joke book* (3rd ed.). Minneapolis, MN: Highbridge Publishing.

Losh, M., Adolphs, R., Poe, M.D., Couture, S., Penn, D., Baranek, G.T., et al. (2009). Neuropsychological profile of autism and the broad autism phenotype. *Archives of General Psychiatry, 66*(5), 518–526.

Miles, J.H., Takahashi, T.N., Bagby, S., Sahota, P.K., Vaslow, D.F., Wang, C.H., et al. (2005). Essential versus complex autism: Definition of fundamental prognostic subtypes. *American Journal of Medical Genetics, 135A,* 171–180.

Myhr, G. (1998) Autism and other pervasive developmental disorders: Exploring the dimensional view. *Canadian Journal of Psychiatry, 43*(6): 589–595.

Reynolds, C.R., & Kamphaus, R.W. (2004). *Behavior Assessment System for Children–2 (BASC-2).* San Antonio, TX: Pearson Publishing.

Scahill, L., McDougle, C.J., Williams, S.K., Dimitropoulos, A., Aman, M.G., McCracken, J.T., et al. (2006). Children's Yale-Brown Obsessive Compulsive Scale modified for pervasive developmental disorders. *Journal of the Academy of Child and Adolescent Psychiatry, 45*(9), 1114–1123.

Thompson, T. (2007). *Making sense of autism.* Baltimore: Paul H. Brookes Publishing Co.

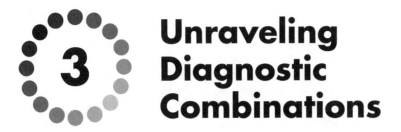

Unraveling Diagnostic Combinations

"In considering any complex matter, we ought to examine every distinct ingredient in the composition, one by one; and reduce everything to the utmost simplicity."

—Edmund Burke, *On Taste* (1756/1909)

We unravel yarn, poetic symbolism, and scientific mysteries. Children with autism are a complex web of traits, abilities, quirks, disabilities, and sometimes disorders that also call for unraveling, at least if we hope to devise ways to help plan a better future for them. This chapter is devoted to unraveling common diagnostic combinations in which autism is one component.

Autism exists as a distinct family of conditions, but the diagnostic process can be confusing. Deciding upon the most appropriate intervention is complicated by the fact that autism and other conditions can coexist in the same person. In the following sections, I discuss some of the conditions that most commonly coexist with ASDs and ways in which intervention can be addressed to those conditions. The unique combination of specific social and communication deficits, as well as the tendency to engage in nonfunctional, repetitive, compulsive behavioral routines, defines ASDs. The following conditions overlap with these three clusters of ASD features at times, but their presence does not negate the reality of ASDs.

MULTIPLE DISABILITIES WITHIN A SINGLE CHILD

It is very common for a child with an autism spectrum diagnosis to experience other mental health or developmental challenges. Next we'll look at a case study of a child with ASD and other challenges.

● ● ● ● ● ● ● ● ●

BEN: A CHILD WITH MULTIPLE DISABILITIES

Ben, 5 years old, was brought to the clinic at the Minnesota Early Autism Project to be evaluated as a candidate for intensive early behavioral intervention based on a suspected diagnosis of an ASD. His parents reported that some of his relatives have bipolar disorder, while others have been diagnosed with ADHD. In addition, Ben has a sibling with mild ASD symptoms, and Ben's mother suffers from recurring depression.

When Ben was between 1 and 2 years of age, his parents noticed several things that were different about him compared with other children his age. He seldom oriented toward his parents when they spoke to him. He didn't show interest in other children. He babbled quite late and began talking at around 16 months of age. When he began talking, he spoke in one- to three-word utterances, using more advanced vocabulary than would be expected for his age. At times, he repeated the same words and phrases over and over, regardless of the situation, and didn't seem to notice whether people were listening to what he said. He stared at objects oddly for extended time intervals. His eye contact was fleeting, and he engaged in intensely repetitive routines such as lining up his toy animals. He descended into tantrums if his compulsive rituals were interrupted. Collectively, Ben exhibited most of the common signs of an ASD.

Ben's development was complicated by more than one challenge. By 2 years of age, Ben behaved like a wind-up toy from the moment he climbed out of bed in the morning until he collapsed in fitful sleep in the evening. He was a nonstop blur of motion—running, jumping, and climbing on and under furniture. He often inadvertently knocked items off shelves and bumped into people and objects without noticing, while producing a constant string of loud vocalizations that disturbed others. He was constantly bruising himself by bumping into things. He picked up a toy truck and pushed it around on the floor for 10 to 20 seconds in sporadic, jerky movements, and then threw it down and picked up another toy, repeating the same behavior pattern. When he became bored, he ran around the room, throwing or kicking a ball, an activity he had been repeatedly told was intended for outdoors. Ben's father described him as "in people's faces" a lot of the time, having no sense of personal space.

At 3 years of age, Ben was enrolled in a special education preschool classroom. His teacher expressed concern that periodically Ben appeared withdrawn and irritable. During those episodes, he played alone and became explosively angry if encroached upon by another child. He cried inexplicably and could not be consoled. He began saying repeatedly that he was a "bad boy" and that he wanted to hurt someone. These episodes lasted for several days or weeks, and then Ben reverted to his nonstop, high-energy activity level. Most of the negative statements disappeared, at least until the next withdrawal episode. Ben's parents and teachers were unable to find anything triggering these unpredictable mood and activity changes, and they were increasingly concerned about Ben.

Ben was evaluated at a multidisciplinary pediatric and psychology clinic, and his symptoms were consistent with the diagnostic criteria for Asperger Disorders and ADHD combined type (Reiff & Tippins, 2004). He was both excessively active and very inattentive, and his intellectual functioning was above the average neurotypical range. The evaluating psychologist said that Ben's moodiness, vacillations from hyperactivity to social isolation, negative self-statements, and anger outbursts could be indications of early stages of bipolar disorder, which was consistent with his family history. She said that it was possible that in a few years Ben may also be diagnosed with Childhood Bipolar Disorder, but that because of his age, she assigned a third diagnosis of Mood Disorder Not Otherwise Specified.

● ● ● ● ● ● ● ● ● ●

Children like Ben pose a diagnostic conundrum for clinicians, therapists, and teachers, who are often unsure where to begin in helping him. Such complex cases are uncommon, but their existence underscores the fact that multiple disabilities can be present within a single child. It is very likely Ben could profit from medication for his ADHD symptoms—such as methylphenidate (Ritalin), dexmethylphenidate (Focalin), or combination amphetamine and dextroamphetamine (Adderall)—and from intensive behavior therapy to overcome his Asperger Disorders symptoms. It is advisable that a child psychiatrist periodically monitors Ben for possible emergence of bipolar disorder symptoms and treat him accordingly should that become necessary.

Ben's case study shows the complex interactions of multiple conditions that can exist in various combinations among children with ASDs. The process of winnowing the diagnostic options and developing focused interventions for each condition is at the heart of effective services for children and youth with ASDs. Ben's complex, overlapping conditions do not negate the validity of his Asperger syndrome diagnosis. It is one piece of a complex puzzle. Ben responded well to a combination of stimulant medication and a naturalistic behavior therapy approach. Only time will tell whether his mood disorder symptoms are really secondary to these other challenges or if they are actually an independent disorder.

ATTENTION-DEFICIT/HYPERACTIVITY DISORDER

Approximately half of all children with ASDs also exhibit clinically diagnosable symptoms of ADHD (Rommelse et al., 2009). Although the *DSM-IV-TR* states that ADHD is not to be diagnosed among children with an ASD, as a practical matter many professionals diagnose and treat concurrent ADHD in autism. Figure 3.1 shows a thought map based on descriptors in the test results and files of a child diagnosed with Autistic Disorder who displayed other challenges as well, such as ADHD. The size of the word indicates how frequently the individual word was mentioned in describing the child (i.e., the larger the word the more frequently it was mentioned; see http://www.thinkmap.com). Among children with ASDs who are higher functioning intellectually and who have milder ASD symptoms, whether they also have significant ADHD symptoms can determine the most appropriate behavioral intervention approach. Children

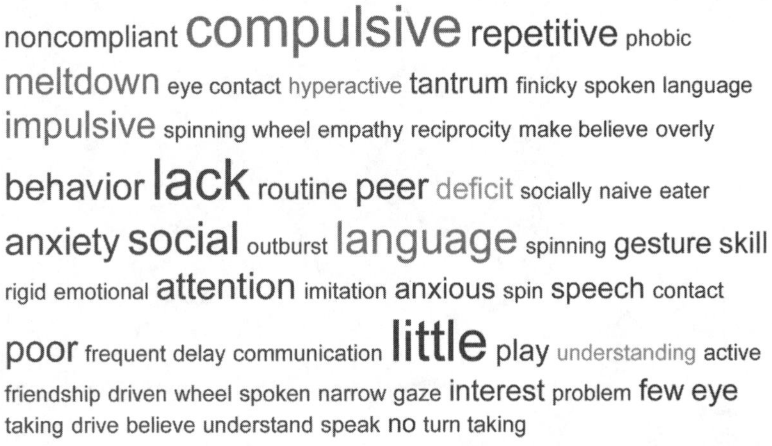

noncompliant **compulsive** repetitive phobic
meltdown eye contact hyperactive **tantrum** finicky spoken language
impulsive spinning wheel empathy reciprocity make believe overly
behavior **lack** routine **peer** deficit socially naive eater
anxiety social outburst **language** spinning **gesture skill**
rigid emotional **attention** imitation **anxious** spin **speech** contact
poor frequent delay communication **little** play understanding active
friendship driven wheel spoken narrow gaze **interest** problem few eye
taking drive believe understand speak no turn taking

Figure 3.1.   A thought map based on descriptors in the test results and files of a child diagnosed with autistic disorder as well as displaying other challenges, like ADHD. The size of the word indicates how frequently the individual word was mentioned in describing the child (the larger the word the more frequently the word is mentioned). Relevance to common daily usage is higher at the bottom of the map than at the top, which tends to involve technical terminology. (Image from the Visual Thesaurus [http://www.visualthesaurus.com], Copyright © 1998–2010 Thinkmap, Inc. All rights reserved; reprinted by permission.)

with ASDs and predominant ADHD symptoms are often noncompliant and can be very difficult to engage in educational activities in school or in home-based therapy. Their behavior is unfocused, erratic, and often disruptive. They often make the greatest progress in a calm, structured environment with minimal distractions. Music, television, computers, and video games should be turned off during interventions and should preferably be in another room. The best initial gains are made when a largely DTI approach is used, interspersed with short periods of free-play activities, even for higher functioning children like Ben. This approach encourages the child to sit in a single setting with minimal distractions and focus his or her attention on specific cues being presented by the teacher or therapist, who systematically rewards the child's responses, small steps toward the educational or therapeutic objective.

Figure 3.2 shows a 5-year-old child participating in naturalistic intervention with a typically developing peer. The therapist has asked the 5-year-old to take turns with her typically developing friend, a skill that is initially lacking among most children with autism.

After the child's behavior is under better instructional or therapeutic control, more naturalistic interventions can be introduced with *higher functioning children,* incorporating interventions within normal daily routines and activities. However, whenever a new, more challenging social or communication skill or other learning task is introduced, it is often wise to revert to a DTI approach until the child has gained confidence and had success with the new challenge. Often if children with ASD and ADHD symptoms are treated with stimulant medications, such as combination amphetamine and dextroamphetamine or methylphenidate, they are more focused and are more responsive to educational or home-based behavior therapy.

These accommodations for a child's ADHD symptoms *should not be used* in place of implementing a typical intensive early behavior therapy strategy that addresses core

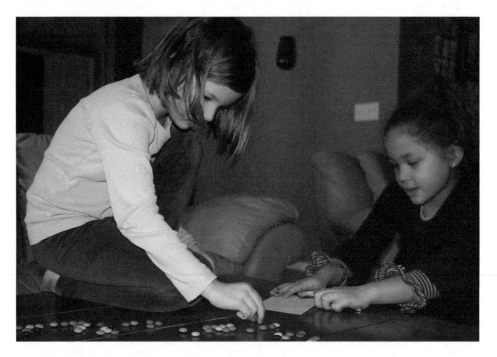

Figure 3.2.   A child with autism (left) with a typically developing peer in a naturalistic (incidental) intervention activity. One of the skills being taught is turn taking.

autism features (i.e., overcoming communication and social skills deficits and compulsive, ritualistic behavior). Both interventions should be implemented conjointly.

ANXIETY DISORDERS

Anxiety and autism go hand in hand (Sinzig, Walter, & Doepfner, 2009; White, Oswald, Ollendick, & Scahill, 2009). Although most children with ASDs exhibit some anxiety problems, for others anxiety is a predominant feature. Social anxiety (e.g., social phobia) and obsessive-compulsive disorder (OCD) are among the most common anxiety problems in autism. Children with ASDs tend to have more phobias triggered by specific situations and by medical fears, but fewer fears of harm or injury, compared with other children with phobias. Among the most common phobias are fears of feeling unsafe outside the home, of being in a crowd or standing in a line, and of traveling in a bus or automobile (various forms of agoraphobia). Individuals with autism often attempt to avoid those situations, which is probably why the fears, phobias, and anxieties of children with ASDs are closely related to other challenging behaviors that permit them to escape or avoid the fearful situation. That is less so for children with other developmental disabilities or neurotypical peers who also have phobias. If typical peers exhibit behavioral challenges, they are usually unrelated to their fears. Among children with ASDs, meltdowns and aggressive outbursts may result from provocation by a fear-inducing stimulus, such as entering a room of strangers or seeing a needle used in a medical procedure (Evans, Canavera, Kleinpeter, Maccubbin, & Taga, 2005). This is an important distinction, because it suggests that addressing behavioral challenges, such as meltdowns and aggression, may often be most effective when it is focused on the child's phobia.

Phobias can be treated as mental health problems independent of core autism symptoms among children and youth with ASDs. In one study (Shabani & Fisher, 2006), stimulus fading combined with rewarding the child for tolerating successive exposures to the fear-inducing stimulus was used with an adolescent with autism and diabetes who had a needle phobia. In *stimulus fading*, a less threatening version of the stimulus is initially presented, such as a picture of the feared object. During each session, a stimulus more like the actual feared stimulus is presented. In this study, the youth's needle phobia had previously prevented adequate medical monitoring of his blood glucose levels for more than 2 years. Gradually exposing him to the fear-inducing stimulus—and rewarding him for tolerating, seeing, and then touching the feared stimulus—was successful in helping the boy and his caregivers obtain daily blood samples for measuring glucose levels (Shabani & Fisher, 2006). Similar results were obtained with another child who feared other medically related stimuli. The child's successful approach responses to the fear-inducing objects were followed by reinforcement. Eventually he was able to tolerate exposure without attempting to escape. During hospital-based desensitization, the boy was able to encounter previously avoided medical equipment and situations. Parents reported that results were maintained after discharge from the hospital (Ricciardi, Luiselli, & Camare, 2006).

Obsessive-compulsive rituals may be stigmatizing and lead to ridicule. Among school-age children with ASDs, those with predominant OCD symptoms are more often bullied by typical peers (50%) than children with mainly phobic symptoms (23%) (Bejerot & Mortberg, 2009). OCD symptoms are apparently easier targets for teasing and physical provocation than social or other anxieties that may be less obvious to classmates. Working with peers to help them empathize with the target child's OCD problems, together with directly treating the OCD, can eliminate bullying. There are excellent resources for teachers and parents to help their peers better understand class-mates with autism, such as *The Autism Acceptance Book* (Sabin, 2006) and *With Open Arms* (Schlieder, 2007).

Medications and Anxiety Disorders

Many parents are apprehensive about asking their child's pediatrician about psy-chotropic medications to treat their child's anxiety problems. It is true that some of the older antipsychotic drugs prescribed many years ago produced bad side effects, like movement disorder or other neurological symptoms. Today, most of the medicines used to treat anxiety problems have relatively mild and limited side effects (many peo-ple experience minimal or no side effects), and they can be very helpful in reducing phobias and obsessive-compulsive symptoms. The most widely used class of drugs are called *selective serotonin reuptake inhibitors* (SSRIs), which were originally developed as an-tidepressants but also have antianxiety properties. The more common are fluoxetine (Prozac); fluvoxamine (Luvox), paroxetine (Paxil), sertraline (Zoloft), and citalopam (Celexa; Kolevzon, Mathewson, & Hollander, 2006).

A 5-year-old boy with PDD-NOS with whom we worked was preoccupied with garage doors. He found it very difficult to concentrate on anything else, because he was obsessed with finding pictures of garage doors in magazines and television ads, and opening and closing the family's garage door repeatedly. When he was prescribed flu-oxetine, most of his perseverative behavior stopped. Such medication treatments are combined with behavioral interventions to promote adaptive skills. A disadvantage of SSRI medications is that, for some children, they can cause insomnia, agitation, and in-creased aggression during the first 2 weeks of treatment or following a dosage increase. Typically, over several weeks, these side effects subside.

OPPOSITIONAL DEFIANT DISORDER

The mother of a 4½-year-old with PDD-NOS said, "You won't believe what Coty did last night when I was on the phone! I was talking with my sister and Coty kept yelling, tug-ging at me, and interrupting. After a few minutes when I hung up the phone, I went in the living room and discovered he had gotten a bottle of chocolate syrup out of the re-frigerator and poured it all over the carpeting." Another mother of a 3 year, 3 month old, also with PDD-NOS, reported that her son, Dylan, screamed, cried, and hit when she asked him to turn off a YouTube *Transformers* video he had already watched repeat-edly for the past 15 minutes. She told him to stop screaming, which seemed to make matters worse. When that didn't produce the result he was seeking (i.e., allowing him to watch the video again), he began abusing their pet dog, yanking its ears and tail, re-quiring her to immediately turn her attention to him. She scolded and tried to reason with Dylan that it was wrong to treat their dog so terribly, but he grinned and tried to turn on the computer video again. She said Dylan's defiant behavior had grown intol-erable to the entire family.

Among the most common parental concerns and complaints regarding their child with autism is the youngster's noncompliant and, at times, openly defiant behavior, as in the examples of Coty and Dylan. Although most children with ASDs are not willfully disobedient, a subset of youngsters with ASDs learn to use defiance as a means of de-manding parental (or teacher) attention. To be diagnosed with *oppositional defiant disor-der* (ODD), the child must exhibit a combination of several characteristics, including negativistic, angry, and defiant behavior lasting for several months, during which time a number of the following are seen:

- The child often loses his or her temper and argues with parents, therapists, or teachers
- The child is easily annoyed by others and appears resentful much of the time
- The child often refuses to comply with adults' requests or rules that are well within his or her ability and may be openly defiant ("You can't make me!")
- The youngster appears to knowingly provoke other people, such as parents or siblings (e.g., by turning up the volume on the television so it is painfully loud)
- The child tends to blame others for his mistakes, and is often spiteful (APA, 2000).

These characteristics are often only seen in higher functioning verbal children with ASDs, are nearly always socially motivated, and are a means of controlling adult behavior. I have known children who are so demanding of adult attention that their mother cannot use the bathroom without allowing the child in the restroom as well. At times, the child may engage in destructive or harmful behavior, such as scribbling on walls with a felt-tip pen or breaking fragile items, in order to command parental attention.

If reasoning with the child or student were effective in resolving the problem, he or she would likely have stopped the behavioral outbursts a long time ago. Parents generally assume scolding is a form of punishment, but for most children with ODD as well as autism, it serves as a powerful reward, even when done with a stern voice. Children with ASDs and ODD seldom show signs of empathy or remorse, which can be doubly difficult for parents and teachers. However, after weeks or months of behavioral intervention, many youngsters appear contrite when they occasionally behave inappropriately, but not always.

Intervention involves a combination of frequent reinforcement for helpful, compliant behavior, while using mild time-outs for ODD behavior. A time-out can be as simple as placing the child on a chair in the corner of the same room, during which time he or she is ignored. I encourage parents or teachers to place a distinctively colored rug under the chair to emphasize the fact that this is a distinct place. Some parents call it the child's "naughty chair." A cooking timer is set for 3 minutes. If the child bolts out of the chair or screams, the timer is reset to 3 minutes and the parent or teacher points to the chair, guides the child back into the chair, and says, "Time-out: When the bell rings you can get up." Nothing else is said. The secret in making this work is that *the child's obstreperous behavior must be absolutely, totally, completely ignored by everyone.* No exceptions, not even for a few seconds. Make no eye contact, don't laugh or smile as a result of any of the child's behavior. Any reaction will tend to perpetuate the child's behavior. That means not looking at the child to see if he or she is feeling unhappy (he or she probably is unhappy) or talking with him or her when they are in the time-out chair. When the child screams, makes loud objections, or threatens, look away and busy yourself with something else. You will probably feel so angry or upset that the hair will stand up on the back of your neck, but you can do it! You really can. It will be very tempting to cajole, coax, wheedle, barter, or otherwise try to help the child (and you) end the unpleasantness. Don't do it! A single episode in which you give in by paying attention to the child's disruptive behavior will require you start the entire process over again, and it will take longer the next time, and even longer the time after that.

When the 3 minutes have elapsed and the child has remained quietly in the chair, nothing is said about the misbehavior at that moment, and the child is encouraged to engage in positive educational or therapeutic activities. Remember, reprimanding the child, or insisting he or she apologize, amounts to giving attention for the very behavior you are trying to reduce. Coercing the child into apologizing often triggers another outburst. If you want to discuss the problem behavior with him or her, wait until both you and the child are calm and pleasantly engaged. Then, you can suggest what your child can do the next time he or she is frustrated and wants your immediate attention, instead of hitting or behaving destructively. Then you can ask him or her to apologize to the person they offended, hit, or shoved. Many children with autism fail to internalize moral lessons about their own inappropriate behavior, though some higher functioning children may be preoccupied with perceived fairness with respect to *others' behavior* (why their brother wasn't punished for a perceived infraction).

In most instances, the foregoing strategy can be combined with a naturalistic incidental teaching or therapy approach, and if applied consistently, the ODD behavior can usually be eliminated within several weeks. Some people will find the child's behavior exceedingly annoying and even offensive, and may say, "He's just spoiled." That is unhelpful and overly simplistic. The presence of ODD and its associated behavior does not indicate that the child's Asperger syndrome or PDD-NOS is fictional or irrelevant. It means the child has two concurrent conditions, both requiring intervention.

Medications for Oppositional Defiant Disorder

There are no specific medications for ODD among children with autism. Among the more commonly prescribed medications are low doses of blood pressure drugs with mild calming effects, such as atenolol (Tenormin) or clonidine (Catapres) (Ming, Gordon, Kang, & Wagner, 2008). Parents sometimes describe their effects as "taking the edge off," but the medications alone seldom eliminate the problem. For some older youngsters with autism and ODD who exhibit aggression, destructiveness, or self-injury, doctors may prescribe atypical antipsychotic medications, such as aripiprazole (Abilify), for a month or two to assist in bringing the behavior under control (Owen et al., 2009). Atypical antipsychotic medications tend to cause weight gain and can increase the risk of Type 2 Diabetes in individuals who may already be at risk, so they are seldom given for prolonged periods to young children. Older children with autism and intellectual disabilities have been treated with mood disorder/seizure medications carbamazepine (Tegretol) or valproic acid (Depakote), though their effects are often unpredictable and they can have significant side effects (Gerstner, et al., 2007; Hellings et al., 2005). In most cases, the most effective interventions are behavioral.

SPEECH-LANGUAGE DISORDERS

Problems with communication are a fundamental feature of ASDs. *Communication* refers to exchange of information between individuals through a common system of symbols, signs, or behavior (Merriam-Webster, 2010). Communication typically involves the use of abstract symbols, such as speech sounds or written symbols, to represent ideas or information exchanged with another person. Communication is not the same as *speech*. Some people communicate with manual signs, others with Picture Exchange Communication System (PECS; Bondy & Frost, 1994) symbols, and others using keyboarding devices. Speech is a specific type of communication that can be dysfunctional among children with autism, but it can also be impaired among neurotypical peers.

Children with autism can have several types of communication problems (American Speech-Language-Hearing Association, 2010b). They may not understand or be motivated to communicate with others and/or may have difficulty grasping abstract aspects of communication (e.g., figures of speech), which is a *pragmatic communication problem*. They may have difficulty coordinating the movements of muscles in their mouth and tongue while expelling air from their lungs in order to make speech sounds, which is a *speech problem* (e.g., apraxia of speech). Finally, they may have a *language impairment*—a particular difficulty with structural aspects of language, such as the distribution and patterning of words, rules governing pronunciation, and arrangement of different types of words in sentences (e.g., *specific language impairment* [SLI]). Nearly all children and youth with autism have pragmatic communication limitations, which is part and parcel of having an ASD. However, in addition, some children with autism have speech problems or language impairments.

In one study, groups of children with SLIs and ASDs, or autism alone, who were matched for nonverbal IQ, were compared for autism spectrum symptoms using standardized autism diagnostic tests. The goal was to determine whether SLI and autism are connected and if the severity of language impairment is correlated with the severity of autism symptoms. There was no relation between the severity of language deficits exhibited by the children with SLI and their scores on the autism diagnostic tests. This seems to indicate that, although there may be some overlap in social and communicative deficits between autism and SLI, they are not the same thing (Leyfer, Tager-Flusberg, Dowd, Tomblin, & Folstein, 2008).

Early Intensive Behavioral Intervention (EIBI) for youngsters with ASDs can improve children's pragmatic communication. It promotes appropriate use of language through teaching multiple exemplars under a range of circumstances, with multiple communication partners, including responding to abstract relationships. However, a child who has speech problems, such as *apraxia of speech* (American Speech-Language-Hearing Association, 2010a), requires the attention of a speech therapist trained in working with children with autism. Typically, speech therapists work with the child on oral-motor exercises as well as producing reliable speech sounds through repetitive practice. Similarly, a child with an ASD who has an SLI is unlikely to overcome that limitation through the use of early intensive behavior intervention alone. By combining forces with a speech-language pathologist who is experienced in treating children with an SLI, behavior therapists and special education teachers can assist the child in prevailing over their language limitation. Behavior therapy staff can often incorporate components of speech therapy prescribed by a speech-language pathologist within ongoing behavior therapy activities by working in close collaboration with the speech clinician.

SUMMARY

It is tempting at times for parents to conclude that a child who displays obstreperous, troubling behavior is "just spoiled" or that she "just wants her way," and that this behavior can be overcome with spanking. Among children with ASDs, that is usually a mistaken interpretation and may backfire. Although a child may have some characteristics that are different from autism, it doesn't mean that the youngster doesn't have autism. Unraveling the complex interactions among multiple conditions that a child with an ASD may experience is an important, but often daunting, aspect of effective intervention. Differential diagnostic assessment designed to sort out exactly which conditions a child has can be time consuming, and it requires an experienced, skilled clinician. Behavioral, social, and communicative interventions for attention, anxiety, speech-language, and oppositional conditions can, at times, be supplemented with appropriate medication. Medications alone are rarely the solution. Taking the time to figure out what you are treating is the first step.

REFERENCES

American Psychiatric Association. (2000). 313.81 Oppositional Defiant Disorder. *Diagnostic and statistical manual of mental disorders* (4th ed., text rev., pp. 100–102). Washington, DC: Author.

American Speech-Language-Hearing Association. (2010a). *Apraxia of speech.* Retrieved April 6, 2010, from http://www.asha.org/slp/clinical/apraxia.htm

American Speech-Language-Hearing Association. (2010b). *Autism (autism spectrum disorders).* Retrieved April 6, 2010, from http://www.asha.org/public/speech/disorders/Autism.htm

Bejerot, S., & Mortberg, E. (2009). Do autistic traits play a role in the bullying of obsessive-compulsive disorder and social phobia sufferers? *Psychopathology, 42,* 170–184.

Bondy, A., & Frost, L. (1994). The Picture Exchange Communication System. *Focus on Autistic Behavior, 9,* 1–19.

Burke, E. (1756/1909). Preface. *On taste* (vol. 24, pt. 1) [Electronic version]. New York: P.F. Collier & Son. Retrieved April 5, 2010, from www.bartleby.com/24/1/

Evans, D.W., Canavera, K., Kleinpeter, F.L., Maccubbin, E., & Taga, K. (2005). The fears, phobias and anxieties of children with autism spectrum disorders and Down syndrome: Comparisons with developmentally and chronologically age matched children. *Child Psychiatry and Human Development, 36,* 3–26.

Gerstner, T., Busing, D., Bell, N., Longin, E., Kasper, J.M., Klostermann, W., et al. (2007). Valproic acid-induced pancreatitis: 16 new cases and a review of the literature. *Journal of Gastroenterology, 42(1),* 39–48.

Hellings, J.A., Weckbaugh, M., Nickel, E.J., Cain, S.E., Zarcone, J.R., Reese, R.M., et al. (2005). A double-blind, placebo-controlled study of valproate for aggression in youth with pervasive developmental disorders. *Journal of Child and Adolescent Psychopharmacology, 15,* 682–692.

Kolevzon, A., Mathewson, K.A., & Hollander, E. (2006). Selective serotonin reuptake inhibitors in autism: A review of efficacy and tolerability. *Journal of Clinical Psychiatry, 67*(3), 407–414.

Leyfer, O.T., Tager-Flusberg, H., Dowd, M., Tomblin, J.B., & Folstein, S.E. (2008). Overlap between autism and specific language impairment: Comparison of Autism Diagnostic Interview and Autism Diagnostic Observation Schedule scores. *Autism Research, 1,* 284–296.

Merriam-Webster. (2010). Communication. In *Merriam-Webster Online Dictionary.* Retrieved April 6, 2010, from http://www.merriam-webster.com/dictionary/communication

Ming, X., Gordon, E., Kang, N., & Wagner, G.C. (2008). Use of clonidine in children with autism spectrum disorders. *Brain Development, 30,* 454–460.

Owen, R., Sikich, L., Marcus, R.N., Corey-Lisle, P., Manos, G., McQuade, R.D., et al. (2009). Aripiprazole in the treatment of irritability in children and adolescents with autistic disorder. *Pediatrics, 124,* 1533–1540.

Reiff, M.I., & Tippins, S. (2004). *ADHD: A complete and authoritative guide.* Elk Grove Village, IL: American Academy of Pediatrics.

Ricciardi, J.N., Luiselli, J.K., & Camare, M. (2006). Shaping approach responses as intervention for specific phobia in a child with autism. *Journal of Applied Behavior Analysis, 39,* 445–448.

Rommelse, N.N., Altink, M.E., Fliers, E.A., Martin, N.C., Buschgens, C.J., Hartman, C.A., et al. (2009). Comorbid problems in ADHD: Degree of association, shared endophenotypes, and formations of distinct subtypes. Implications for future DSM. *Journal of Abnormal Child Psychology, 37,* 793–804.

Sabin, E. (2006). *The autism acceptance book.* New York: Watering Can Press.

Schlieder, M. (2007). *With open arms: Creating school communities of support for kids with social challenges using circle of friends, extracurricular activities, and learning teams.* Shawnee Mission, KS: Autism Asperger Publishing.

Shabani, D.B., & Fisher, W. (2006). Stimulus fading and differential reinforcement for the treatment of needle phobia in a youth with autism. *Journal of Applied Behavior Analysis, 39,* 449–452.

Sinzig, Walter, & Doepfner. (2009). Attention deficit/hyperactivity disorder in children and adolescents with autism spectrum disorder: Symptom or syndrome? *Journal of Attention Disorders, 13,* 117–126.

Unwin, G.L., & Deb, S. (2008). Use of medication for the management of behavior problems among adults with intellectual disabilities: a clinicians' consensus survey. *American Journal on Mental Retardation, 113,* 19–31.

White, S.W., Oswald, D., Ollendick, T., & Scahill, L. (2009). Anxiety in children and adolescents with autism spectrum disorders. *Clinical Psychology Review, 219,* 216–229.

Yood, M.U., DeLorenze, G., Quesenberry, C.P., Jr., Oliveria, S.A., Tsai, A.L., Willey, V.J., et al. (2009). The incidence of diabetes in atypical antipsychotic users differs according to agent—Results from a multisite epidemiologic study. *Pharmacoepidemiology and Drug Safety, 18,* 791–799.

4 Predicting Intervention Outcome

"I dwell in possibility."

—Emily Dickinson, *The Complete Poems* (1899/1976)

Physicist Niels Bohr said, "Prediction is very difficult, especially of the future" (Ellis, 1970; p. 431). But, difficult or not, we want to know with some confidence what the outcome is likely to be for a child with autism if we choose one course of intervention over another. Two groups of factors affect both selection and outcomes of autism early intervention: *child characteristics* and *intervention features*. Until recently, little attention was paid to child characteristics as predictors of early intervention results and how those differences might inform the choice of intervention approach. This is the first focus of Chapter 4. Much of the discussion regarding autism early intervention has focused on merits of applied behavior analysis (ABA) versus non-ABA approaches, which has generated more heat than light. Even within ABA approaches, advocates of one versus another method have often engaged in unproductive quarreling about their effectiveness. There have been few comparison studies of the various subtypes of ABA interventions that provide a clear basis for conclusions about the efficacy of one intervention over another. In reality, there are numerous differences among early intervention strategies that may affect outcome, in addition to whether they are based on ABA principles. In this chapter, these differences and their relevance to outcomes are examined.

FACTORS INFLUENCING EARLY INTERVENTION CHOICE AND EFFECTIVENESS

Children's responses to the same therapy approach, including comparable intensity of intervention, can vary widely.

● ● ● ● ● ● ● ● ●

Aaron and Sergio are both 4 years old and diagnosed with ASD. For the past 2 years, they have both received an average of 25–30 hours per week of one-to-one Early Intensive Behavioral intervention (EIBI) employing largely DTI. Aaron is now making spontaneous requests, responding to questions, and initiating conversations with his parents using 3- to 5-word phrases. He is playing reciprocally with same-age typically developing peers, and his compulsive behavior of lining up objects and intently peering at them has largely stopped. Sergio, after the same amount of time receiving EIBI, is making some requests with single-word utterances and using picture symbols to communicate, but most of the time he must be prompted to do so. He engages in some parallel play with same-age peers but no interactive play. He continues to be preoccupied with intensely watching the credits at the end of his favorite cartoon video, repeatedly scanning back and forth on his father's computer. Sergio has periodic meltdowns if he is asked to turn off the computer.

● ● ● ● ● ● ● ● ● ●

Child Characteristics

These differences in Aaron and Sergio's responses to the same overall duration and intensity and method of EIBI seem puzzling, but such an outcome is common. Let's consider some of the factors that account for such differences.

Early Age of Intervention

Though Sergio and Aaron both began receiving therapy around 2 years of age, many children with autism receive few special services until they are 4 or 5 years of age (Lord & McGee, 2001). The age at which a child begins EIBI is correlated with outcome, with earlier entry predictive of a better outcome. Worried parents of a 5½-year-old who had received no previous early intervention services asked me, " Is it too late for our daughter?" My heart went out to them. "Not at all," I replied. "It is likely a child who is between 5 and 6 years old when she first begins EIBI will make significant gains, but the amount of improvement may be somewhat less than a child who is 2 or 3 years old when beginning intervention." It is also possible that similar improvements may be achieved, but more slowly and laboriously.

Social Interest

A child's social interest and responsiveness is one of the most important factors predicting a favorable outcome of EIBI. By 1 month after birth, typically developing infants can maintain eye contact; by 2 months, they smile and coo in response to others; and by 3 months, they babble, giggle, and laugh when an adult plays with them, and show surprise, happiness, and fear. Between 6 and 9 months, most infants respond by turning to look when their name is called, and begin to enjoy Peek-a-boo and Pat-a-cake games. About this same age, babies begin to reach out with their hands for familiar people to hold them. They may also become fearful of strangers.

Many children who are later diagnosed with an ASD show few, if any, of these typical social developmental signs in their first year or two of life. Children with autism who display some of these social responses by age 2 have a better prognosis in early intervention than those who exhibit few, if any, of them. The more socially responsive by age 2, the more likely a child may profit from naturalistic intervention. Children who are more socially responsive are better candidates for Blended and Incidental Interventions (Stahmer, Schreibman & Cunningham, 2010).

Joint Attention

Joint attention in early childhood falls into two categories, revealed by a child's responses to attempts of others to get his or her attention or the child's spontaneous initiations. *Responding to joint attention* refers to infants' ability to follow the direction of the gaze and gestures of others in order to share a common point of reference.

Alternatively, *initiating joint attention* involves the child's use of gestures and eye contact to direct others' attention to objects, events, and themselves. Children initiating joint attention show or spontaneously share their interests or pleasurable experiences with others (Mundy & Newall, 2007). Joint attention typically develops around age 1 and is important in building social connections. Before age 1, infants merely look at the hand of the person pointing, whereas later they look in the direction of the pointing, called a *distal point*. Joint attention provides a reason for the child to pay attention to social cues provided by others, because the child obtains useful information (e.g., something's location). The presence of some joint attention is predictive of a better outcome in EIBI, especially naturalistic interventions. The more complex a child's display of joint attention, the better the likely outcome.

Social Referencing

Social referencing refers to the child's ability to observe a parent's emotional response to an ambiguous situation (e.g., a stranger who enters the room or a novel object that appears in the room) as a means of determining whether the new thing or person is potentially harmful. The parent who looks apprehensive signals to the child that the new person or object may be harmful. That process begins around age 6 months and continues to around age 2 (Walden & Ogan, 1988). Children with an autism spectrum diagnosis who engage in some social referencing have better prognosis in EIBI, especially children receiving naturalistic interventions.

Language

Children who say some words at the time they begin EIBI have a better prognosis than those who do not. Even if the child says words repetitively and nonfunctionally (called *echolalia*), that is predictive of a better outcome than if he or she says no words. For example, echolalia was found to be predictive of a more positive response to Pivotal Response Treatment (PRT; Schreibman, Stahmer, Barlett, & Dufek, 2009; Sherer & Schreibman, 2005). Functional use of words or short phrases, such as making requests, augurs well for how a child is likely to respond to naturalistic interventions.

Imitation

The single best predictor at age 2 of a positive social outcome at age 6 or 7 resulting from EIBI is motor or verbal imitation. The correlation was high (i.e., .91) in the Sallows and Graupner (2005) study. Motor imitation requires a functioning brain *mirror neuron* system, which is thought to be related to empathy (Gazzola, Aziz-Zadeh, & Keysers, 2006; Iacoboni, 2009). Mirror neurons are nerve cells that respond to seeing someone else perform an action (e.g., reaching), much as if the observer had performed the action her- or himself. They mirror the observed person's action.

Anxiety/Fearfulness

Nearly every child with an ASD experiences more anxiety or fearfulness challenges than their same-age typical peers. Some are extreme, including phobic rejection of any new person, activity, or object that might be part of intervention. Others' fears are limited to unfamiliar social situations, which are very common. Finally, many children on the autism spectrum worry about being unable to engage in their highly preferred compulsive routines, like lining up objects, opening and closing doors, or flipping light switches. Children with extreme phobic reactions to any novel stimulus, including other people, are generally poor candidates for an Incidental Intervention approach, which is generally too unpredictable for their comfort level. Children who are worried about being unable to carry out their rituals can often have their fears assuaged by being provided brief access to their routines after completing tasks. Over time, as they become more comfortable and trusting of therapists or teachers, their anxiety generally subsides. Generally, the more fearful a child is at intervention entry, the more structured the intervention needs to be. Highly fearful children may adapt more quickly to DTI, but children with more joint attention and early language skills may profit from making the transition to Blended Intervention.

Stereotypic and Ritualistic Behavior

Children who engage in more hand-flapping, twirling, rocking, or repetitive compulsive routines are generally less socially responsive and are more likely to be inflexible. These characteristics, especially in combination with lower cognitive ability, are associated with a less favorable intervention outcome. Stereotypic, compulsive behaviors indicate a child with an ASD is more likely to be responsive to DTI than an Incidental Intervention approach. Some children with these characteristics may profit from a Blended Intervention, beginning with DTI and fading to more naturalistic strategies as the repetitive nonfunctional behavior subsides.

Attention-Deficit/Hyperactivity Disorder Symptoms

The more symptoms a child with ASD has that conform to those of ADHD, the slower his or her progress in early intervention. A child with 4 to 6 of 15 possible ADHD symptoms is generally not a good candidate for a naturalistic intervention approach. Greater cognitive ability can compensate in part for ADHD symptoms, but only up to a point. Such children generally require more structure and procedural consistency than are part of an Incidental Intervention approach. Higher functioning children with ASDs may profit from a Blended Intervention, beginning with more structure and fading to an Incidental Intervention approach.

Autism Intervention Responsiveness Scale

Figure 4.1, the Autism Intervention Responsiveness Scale (AIRS™), Research Edition, shows the relationship between child characteristics and types of interventions that are likely to be effective for a given child. The first vertical column lists major child factors, or domains that differ among children. Raters are to look at the descriptions of behaviors being exhibited for each domain and indicate how closely those behaviors match those of the child with the corresponding number in the far-left column. They then assign a numerical rating to each child domain (1 to 3), sum all ratings for the child, and divide by 12, yielding an average rating from 1.0 to 3.0. Children scoring 1.0–1.49 are likely candidates for DTI, whereas those scoring 2.5–3.0 will likely profit from Incidental Intervention. Children whose average ratings are 1.5–2.49 will likely make the most rapid and consistent gains with a Blended Intervention approach. Those scoring 1.5–1.99 may require DTI intervention to begin therapy for the first month or two, and may continue to require a DTI strategy whenever a new goal is introduced. Those

Autism Intervention
Responsiveness Scale (AIRS™)

Instructions: The AIRS form is to be completed by raters who are parents or other caregivers who have devoted a minimum of 20 hours with the child within the preceding 2-week period. Raters are expected to be familiar with the meaning of such autism developmental terms as *joint attention, imitation,* and *insistence on sameness.* For each domain raters are to print the numerical rating (1, 2, or 3) in the domain rating (right-hand column).

Domain	1	2	3	Domain rating
Communication (COM)	Does not speak or use gestures to communicate; may exhibit nonfunctional vocalizations or repetitive words	Uses spoken single words or phrases and some gestures to communicate; follows single-step instructions	Considerable phrase speech; tendency for excessive verbosity; follows multistep instructions	
Joint Attention (JAT)	No Joint Attention	Some or occasional Joint Attention	Frequent Joint Attention	
Imitation (IMT)	No motor or verbal imitation	Some motor and limited verbal imitation	Good motor and moderate to good verbal imitation	
Social Interest (SNT)	Shows no interest in people except to meet his or her needs; prefers to be left alone	Some social interest but lacks skills to interact with others	Definite social interest; prefers to be with other people, but lacks typical social skills	
Insistence on Sameness (INS)	Many activities performed as rigid daily routines; tantrums if routines are not followed	Appears uncomfortable if predictable routines are not followed, but tolerates some changes	Has one or two highly specific routines (e.g., bedtime), but otherwise flexible about daily activities	
Narrow Interests (NIT)	Interested in 1–3 toys or motor activities; no interest in purposeful games; motor activities are performed with little variability	Interested in several toys or activities or games, but can be distracted fairly easily to engage with another toy or activity	Interested in specific verbal topics (e.g., dinosaurs, vehicles, weather), computer games, or complex toys; can be distracted verbally; may resist or protest	

(continued)

AIRS™

Figure 4.1. Autism Intervention Responsiveness Scale (AIRS™), Research Edition.

Autism Intervention Responsiveness Scale (AIRS™) *(continued)*

Domain	1	2	3	Domain rating
Repetitive Motor Behavior (RMB)	Nearly constant nonfunctional repetitive motor behavior involving body parts, items of clothing, thread, or a single toy; extremely difficult to redirect	Moderate repetitive motor behavior, but can be distracted by another activity; motor behavior involves parts of the environment, such as light switches, doors, videos, vehicles	Infrequent, brief, mild self-stimulatory motor behavior when excited or upset; otherwise no stereotypic mannerisms	
Intellectual Ability (INT)	IQ < 60	IQ 60–84	IQ 85 or above	
Attention (ATT)	Fleeting, very poor attention	Fair to moderate attention to tasks	Attends to tasks for extended period	
Activity (ACT)	Nearly constantly moving; does not persist at any activity more than seconds	More active than same-age typical peers; sits still for several minutes to participate in some activities	Generally calm, readily remains seated; does not appear more active than typical peers	
Anxiety/ Fearfulness (ANX)	Often fearful in many situations	Moderate anxiety in several situations	Not overly apprehensive; exhibits anxiety in novel situations	
Physical Features (PHS)	Atypically small or large head size; atypical teeth spacing/size, ear features, or eye/brow placement; other unusual physical features	Subtle difference in some facial features from others, but not strikingly unusual appearance; normal head size	Typical features resembling those of other family members and typical peers; normal head size	
Sum of Individual Scale Ratings				

Scoring: Overall AIRS Rating is obtained by summing individual scale ratings (1 + 2 + 3) divided by 12 = Mean AIRS Rating. Each domain rating is a Likert item, the sum of which yields a Likert Scale Score.

AIRS Ratings Interpretation: Child will most likely make greatest developmental gains from:

1.0–1.49: Discrete Trial Intervention alone

1.5–1.99: Beginning with Discrete Trial Intervention and slow transition to some Incidental Interventions

2.0–2.49: Beginning with Discrete Trial Intervention followed by transition to mostly Incidental Interventions

2.5–3.0: Incidental Teaching/Therapy alone

AIRS Profile

- -

Instructions: For each domain, raters mark an X in the box corresponding to the average score for that domain. The first seven scales—COM through RMB—are core autism symptoms. The five scales indicated in gray (INT through PHS) are factors that moderate expression of autism symptoms. The pattern of scores on the first seven scales indicates severity of autism symptoms and factors that will moderate expression of those symptoms (last 5 scales). When most domain ratings fall in the 1.0–1.49 range, that generally indicates severe autism symptoms; 1.5–2.49 indicates severe to moderate symptoms, and 2.5–3.0 indicates moderate to mild autism symptoms. Children for which most domain scores fall in the 1.5–2.49 range who also have scores of 1.0–2.0 on INT, ATT, ACT, ANX, or PHS are likely to have greater challenges than children with similar core autism symptom scores with moderator scale scores of 2.5–3.0. Intervening to address ATT, ANX, and ACT and improving language skills may reduce core autism symptoms.

- -

AIRS Profile:

Domain	COM	JAT	IMT	SNT	INS	NIT	RMB	INT	ATT	ACT	ANX	PHS
2.5–3.0												
2.0–2.49												
1.5–1.99												
1.0–1.49												

who score 2.00–2.49 will likely profit from participation in DTI for a lesser amount of time with more rapid transition to Incidental Intervention.

This tool is intended to assist the reader in thinking about planning interventions based on child characteristics and is not intended to be strictly prescriptive. It is purely a heuristic for thinking about the range of intervention options and their integration to best match a child's needs. In evaluating which type, combination, and intensity of intervention is most effective for a given child, the intervention team is responsible for closely monitoring child progress under each intervention condition.

Intervention Features

Proponents of one early intervention approach versus another often point out that the methods they are advocating grow out of a specific theory of child development or learning. In reality, despite theoretical differences, early intervention methods often share significant features in common (e.g., following the child's lead is common to PRT, Floortime, and Incidental Intervention) but may differ widely in other respects, not necessarily having very much to do with their preferred theory. In this section I will examine some factors that have been shown to affect child outcomes of EIBI.

Applied Behavior Analysis Principles

Although early intervention methods based on ABA principles are widely recognized as effective (e.g., Lord & McGee, 2001; National Autism Center, 2009; Sallows & Graupner, in press), other approaches to early intervention are used as well. Several emphasize developmentally coordinated emotional self-regulation; age-appropriate cognitive experiences; and, perhaps most important, the parent–child relationship as the centerpiece of intervention (e.g., Greenspan's [2006] Floortime and Gutstein & Sheely's [2002] Relationship Development Intervention). The Early Start Denver Model developed by Geraldine Dawson, Sally Rogers, and colleagues (2010) employs coordinated, interactive social interactions focusing on imitation and symbolic and interpersonal (nonverbal, affective, pragmatic) communication. In addition, teaching occurs to overcome the learning deficits that have resulted from the child's past lack of access to the social world due to the effects of autism. The SCERTS® Model (Prizant, Wetherby, Rubin, Laurent, & Rydell, 2005), originally developed by Prizant and Wetherby, builds competence in social communication, emotion regulation, and transactional support through a complex set of assessment-based interventions. *Transactional supports* refer to environmental adaptations based on specific child needs and characteristics.

One of the more widely used early intervention and school-based approaches that *does not* rely on ABA principles is the Treatment and Education of Autistic and Communication-Related Handicapped Children (TEACCH) program developed by Eric Schopler (Mesibov, Shea, & Schopler, 2004). It is based on theories of cognitive and emotional development, and includes a combination of physical structure, scheduling, a work system to indicate expectations, a transportable routine, and visual structure.

Parents, teachers, and therapists often have difficulty evaluating which type of early intervention is most effective for a particular child. In 2001 a committee of the National Research Council, chaired by Catherine Lord and James McGee, reviewed all autism early intervention studies through 2000. The committee concluded that the only interventions producing lasting improvements in the core symptoms of autism were based on ABA principles (Lord & McGee, 2001). A subsequent survey was conducted of 25 autism early intervention outcome studies: 20 studies evaluated interventions based on ABA, 3 studies evaluated TEACCH, and 2 studies evaluated the Colorado Health Sciences Model. Outcome studies were graded according to their scientific quality and subsequently evaluated according to the magnitude of results documented in the studies. Using criteria employed in other psychological treatment outcome studies, it was concluded that "Based on these guidelines interventions based on ABA will be considered 'Well Established.'" TEACCH and Colorado Health Science model will be considered neither "Well Established" nor "Probably efficacious" (Eikeseth, 2009). Recently Sallows and Graupner (in press) have exhaustively summarized the autism early intervention literature and arrived at a similar conclusion: The degree to which early interventions employ ABA principles predicts better outcomes. The National Standards Project's (National Autism Center, 2009) evaluative summary of autism interventions indicates various combined behavioral interventions including PRT and TEACCH are effective and considered "established interventions" for many children with ASDs.

Sufficient Intensity

The importance of intensity of a child's early experiences is not specific to ABA therapy and autism. In a landmark study, Betty Hart and Todd Risley (1995) studied language and intellectual development of typically developing preschool children growing up in poor inner-city neighborhoods and others whose parents were middle-class professional families. Although it wasn't surprising that the two groups of children displayed some language differences, what *was* surprising was the *profound differences in the language experience* of the two groups of children and the resulting differences in intellectual and language competence. In a review of the role of intervention intensity in language intervention, Warren, Fey, and Yoder (2007) noted, "Cumulative intervention intensity makes a meaningful difference in language learning." They also emphasized that it isn't always the case that massed trials, as usually occur in DTI, yield superior results to distributed practice even when they have a similar total time in intervention. However, if a child receives 30 hours per week of EIBI, it would be difficult to achieve comparable total intervention intensity by spacing intervention episodes farther apart, unless the intervention periods included weekends and evenings.

In a more recent study, Steve Warren and colleagues (Warren et al., 2009) used an automated device to track all utterances of preschool children with autism and those of people around each child, such as parents or therapists. They found that during periods when children with autism were in therapy, the number of the child's total utterances, including conversational exchanges, greatly increased (Figure 4.2). Several studies of ABA-based autism early intervention indicate that engaging in more hours per week of early intervention produces greater improvements in intellectual, language, and social functioning than fewer hours (Cohen, Amerine-Dickens, & Smith, 2006; Eikeseth, Smith, Jahr, & Eldevik, 2002, 2007; Lovaas, 1987). In comparison to the high-intensity studies, several lower intensity intervention programs have also been conducted; while reporting improvements, they generally showed lesser reductions of autism symptoms and skills improvement (Bibby, Eikeseth, Martin, Mudford, & Reeves, 2001; Remington et al., 2007; Smith, Buch, & Gamby, 2000; Smith, Groen, & Wynn, 2000).

Most evidence indicates that 25–30 hours per week of one-to-one intervention over the first 1–2 years is required to make significant gains in core autism symptoms for children who are responsive to this form of intervention (Lord & McGee, 2001). Some parents prefer to begin with 10 to 20 hours of therapy per week and then increase

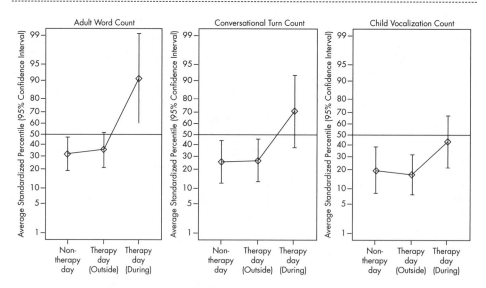

Figure 4.2. Automated language interaction measures among children with autism on non-therapy days, on therapy days outside of therapy, and on therapy days during therapy. Left panel shows total adult verbal counts, middle panel total number of conversational exchanges between child and adult, and right panel total child verbal counts. (From Warren, S.F., Gilkerson, J., Richards, J.A., Oller, D.K., Xu, D., Yapanel, U., et al. [2009]. What automated vocal analysis reveals about the vocal production and language learning environment of young children with autism. *Journal of Autism and Developmental Disorders, 40*[5], 555–569; reprinted with kind permission from Springer Science & Business Media B.V.)

intervention intensity later if the child's gains are judged to be insufficient. It is important to bear in mind that the majority of cognitive, language, and social gains are made in the first 18 months of early intervention (see Figure 2 in Sallows & Graupner, 2005). Increasing intervention intensity after 1 to 2 years may not compensate for *learning that did not occur* during the period when most rapid skill development and brain connectivity normally occur. Providing inadequate intensity during that early period may undermine the purpose of EIBI.

Contextually Nested Interventions

Skills taught out of context may not generalize to natural settings where they are ultimately intended to be displayed. Using stimuli and reinforcers that are unrelated to the context (e.g., tokens instead of natural consequences for requesting a sippy cup of apple juice) is less likely to engender generalization and maintenance once therapy is phased out. Tying a child's verbal or picture symbol requests to their natural consequences, such as a preferred activity, will make it more likely the child will make a similar request under comparable circumstances in the future. Discrete Trial or Incidental Teaching sessions embedded within normal daily routines at school or home are more likely to be adopted by caregivers and to be maintained when specialized instructional or therapy staff are not present. At times it may be necessary to conduct massed therapy or learning trials taught out of context to maintain the child's attention and to teach difficult discriminations. However, when it is possible to do so, capitalizing upon incidental learning opportunities within natural contexts can be highly effective.

Multiple Teachers/Therapists and Multiple Settings

No systematic studies have been reported of the role of multiple teaching or therapy staff across several settings in early intervention programs. In the National Research

Council review (Lord & McGee, 2001), conducting such a study was one of the recommendations. Based on intolerance of children with autism for changes, including interacting with different people, and in order to promote generalization across settings, this is a reasonable recommendation, and one we routinely employ in our early intervention endeavors.

Participation of Siblings and Peers

• • • • • • • • • •

Tobias, who just turned 3 years old, spends Monday, Wednesday, and Friday mornings in a typical preschool classroom. He has been diagnosed with PDD-NOS. He watches two boys playing with cars on a mat in the play area. He approaches them and hesitates. He appears to want to play with the boys, but he doesn't know how to join in. Finally, he kicks a ball so it ricochets across the floor and bangs into the boys' toy cars. They shout at him, "Stop it! Go away!" Tobias runs away crying.

• • • • • • • • • •

Few preschool-age children with autism have the skills to play interactively with same-age peers, other than very simple "chase" or "play fight" games similar to those they see on cartoons. Often siblings learn to accommodate their sister or brother with an ASD, facilitating limited play while at home, but that seldom generalizes to interacting effectively with other children who are less motivated to find ways to be helpful to the child with autism. One approach to encouraging peer-oriented social skills involves nesting intervention within an integrated setting alongside neurotypical peers. Gail McGee's Little Walden program at Emory University (McGee & Morrier, 2009) and Phil Strain's LEAP school-based interventions (Strain, McGee, & Kohler, 2001) explicitly combine children with autism with neurotypical peers in order to promote appropriate social interactions. Although that may be effective for some higher functioning children, in our experience more explicit teaching of basic communication and social skills is necessary to enable most children with autism to initiate and sustain social interactions with peers, including games and toy play. Interventions that explicitly teach interactive play and communication with peers are more likely to have positive outcomes. By all means, typical siblings and peers can be included in carefully crafted social interaction activities with a child or student with an ASD, but don't expect her or him to learn by osmosis to be socially competent.

Proactive Strategies for Preventing Behavioral Challenges

Effective EIBI programs do not wait for behavioral challenges to arise before acting. They anticipate and prevent them. Most behavioral challenges in young children with ASDs are a result of a child's inability to communicate needs and wants, as well as being thwarted in highly preferred activities or access to desired commodities. Proactive strategies that obviate the need for tantrums, aggression, and other emotional/behavioral outbursts can be highly effective (Carr et al., 2002).

SUMMARY

There is currently no foolproof method for predicting a given child's response to various types of EIBI services with a high degree of accuracy. That is not the same as saying we are unable to predict which child and intervention features are likely to yield better outcomes, because we generally can do so. Weighing the degree to which a child exhibits challenges in the following domains can guide the choice of intervention: attention/hyperactivity, anxiety, compulsive behavior, imitation, intellectual functioning, joint attention, language, social interest, social referencing, and stereotypic behavior. In most instances, the relative challenges in the combination of these domains predict whether a Discrete Trial, Blended, or Incidental Intervention is most appropriate.

REFERENCES

Bibby, P., Eikeseth, S., Martin, N.T., Mudford, O.C., & Reeves, D. (2001). Progress and outcomes for children with autism receiving parent-managed intensive interventions. *Research in Developmental Disabilities, 22*(6), 425–447.

Carr, E.G., Dunlap, G., Horner, R.H., Koegel, R.L., Turnbull, A.P., Sailor, W., et al. (2002). Positive behavior support: Evolution of applied science. *Journal of Positive Behavior Interventions, 4*(1), 4–16.

Cohen, H., Amerine-Dickens, M., & Smith, T. (2006). Early intensive behavioral treatment: Replication of the UCLA model in a community setting. *Journal of Developmental and Behavioral Pediatrics, 27*(Suppl. 2), S145–S155.

Dawson, G., Rogers, S., Munson, J., Smith, M., Winter, J., Greenson, J., et al. (2010). Randomized, controlled trial of an intervention for toddlers with autism: The Early Start Denver Model. *Pediatrics, 125*(1), e17–23.

Dickinson, E. (1976). *The complete poems.* London: Faber & Faber. (Original work published 1899)

Eikeseth, S. (2009). Outcome of comprehensive psycho-educational interventions for young children with autism. *Research in Developmental Disabilities, 30*(1), 158–178.

Eikeseth, S., Smith, T., Jahr, E., & Eldevik, S. (2002). Intensive behavioral treatment at school for 4- to 7-year-old children with autism. A 1-year comparison controlled study. *Behavior Modification, 26*(1), 49–68.

Eikeseth, S., Smith, T., Jahr, E., & Eldevik, S. (2007). Outcome for children with autism who began intensive behavioral treatment between ages 4 and 7: A comparison controlled study. *Behavior Modification, 31*(3), 264–278.

Ellis, A.K. (1970). *Teaching and learning elementary social studies.* Boston: Allyn & Bacon.

Gazzola, V., Aziz-Zadeh, L., & Keysers, C. (2006). Empathy and the somatotopic auditory mirror system in humans. *Current Biology, 16*(18), 1824–1829.

Greenspan, S.I. (2006). *Engaging autism: Helping children relate, communicate and think with the DIR Floortime approach.* Cambridge, MA: Da Capo Lifelong Books.

Gutstein, S.E., & Sheely, R.K. (2002). *Relationship development intervention with young children: Social and emotional development activities for Asperger syndrome, autism, PDD and NLD.* London: Jessica Kingsley Publishers.

Hart, B., & Risley, T.R. (1995). *Meaningful differences in the everyday experience of young American children.* Baltimore: Paul H. Brookes Publishing Co.

Iacoboni, M. (2009). Imitation, empathy, and mirror neurons. *Annual Review of Psychology, 60,* 653–670.

Lord, C.E., & McGee, J. (Eds.). (2001). *Educating children with autism.* Division of Behavioral Sciences. National Research Council. Washington, DC: National Academies Press.

Lovaas, O.I. (1987). Behavioral treatment and normal educational and intellectual functioning in young autistic children. *Journal of Consulting and Clinical Psychology, 55*(1), 3–9.

McGee, G.G., & Morrier, M.J. (2009). Combining inclusion and ABA programming: The Walden incidental teaching model and curriculum. *Autism Advocate, 55*(2), 38–42.

Mesibov, G.B., Shea, V., & Schopler, E. (2004). *The TEACCH approach to autism spectrum disorders.* New York: Springer.

Mundy, P., & Newall, L. (2007). Attention, joint attention, and social cognition. *Current Directions in Psychological Science, 16*(5), 269–274.

National Autism Center. (2009). *National standards report. Proceedings from National Standards Project.* Randolph, MA: Author.

Prizant, B.M., Wetherby, A.M., Rubin, E., Laurent, A.C., & Rydell, P.J. (2005). *The SCERTS® Model: A comprehensive educational approach for children with autism spectrum disorders* (Vols. 1–2). Baltimore: Paul H. Brookes Publishing Co.

Remington, B., Hastings, R.P., Kovshoff, H., degli Espinosa, F., Jahr, E., Brown, T., et al. (2007). Early intensive behavioral intervention: Outcomes for children with autism and their parents after two years. *American Journal on Mental Retardation, 112*(6), 418–438.

Rizzolatti, G., & Fabbri-Destro, M. (2010). Mirror neurons: From discovery to autism. *Experimental Brain Research, 200*(3–4), 223–237.

Sallows, G.O., & Graupner, T.D. (2005). Intensive behavioral treatment for children with autism: four-year outcome and predictors. *American Journal on Mental Retardation, 110*(6), 417–438.

Sallows, G.O., & Graupner, T.D. (in press). Autism spectrum disorders. In P. Sturmey and M. Hersen (Eds.), *Handbook of evidence-based practice in clinical psychology: Vol. 1. Child and adolescent disorders* (p. 427). New York: Wiley.

Schreibman, L., Stahmer, A.C., Barlett, V.C., & Dufek, S. (2009). Brief report: Toward refinement of a predictive behavioral profile for treatment outcome in children with autism. *Research on Autism Spectrum Disorders, 3*(1), 163–172.

Sherer, M.R., & Schreibman, L. (2005). Individual behavioral profiles and predictors of treatment effectiveness for children with autism. *Journal of Consulting and Clinical Psychology, 73*(3), 525–538.

Smith, T., Buch, G.A., & Gamby, T.E. (2000). Parent-directed, intensive early intervention for children with pervasive developmental disorder. *Research in Developmental Disabilities, 21*(4), 297–309.

Smith, T., Groen, A.D., & Wynn, J.W. (2000). Randomized trial of intensive early intervention for children with pervasive developmental disorder. *American Journal on Mental Retardation, 105*(4), 269–285.

Stahmer, A.C., Schreibman, L., & Cunningham, A.B. (2010) Toward a technology of treatment individualization for young children. *Brain Research.* doi:10.1016/j.brainres.2010.09.043

Strain, P.S., McGee, G.G., & Kohler, F.W. (2001). Inclusion of children with autism in early intervention: An examination of rationale, myths, and procedures. In M.J. Guralnick (Ed.), *Early childhood inclusion: Focus on change* (pp. 337–363). Baltimore: Paul H. Brookes Publishing Co.

Walden, T.A., & Ogan, T.A. (1988). The development of social referencing. *Child Development, 59*(5), 1230–1240.

Warren, S.F., Fey, M.E., & Yoder, P.J. (2007). Differential treatment intensity research: A missing link to creating optimally effective communication interventions. *Mental Retardation and Developmental Disabilities Research Reviews, 13*(1), 70–77.

Warren, S.F., Gilkerson, J., Richards, J.A., Oller, D.K., Xu, D., Yapanel, U., et al. (2009). What automated vocal analysis reveals about the vocal production and language learning environment of young children with autism. *Journal of Autism and Developmental Disorders, 40*(5), 555–569.

Evidence-Based Practice

"Take nothing on its looks; take everything on evidence. There's no better rule."

Charles Dickens, *Great Expectations* (1861/2008)

When we think of *evidence*, Sherlock Holmes comes to mind. But evidence also refers to information obtained as part of a scientific investigation, whether it is information about the surface of Mars or the behavior of children with autism in home, clinical, or educational settings. This chapter will discuss *evidence-based practice*—the idea that certain treatments, interventions, or methods can be preferred to others based upon research and statistically significant effectiveness.

HOW DO WE DECIDE WHETHER AN INTERVENTION IS EFFECTIVE?

Faith has a 2½-year-old son, Garrett, who was recently diagnosed with Autistic Disorder. After explaining the diagnosis, the child's pediatrician and psychologist said that it was important that Garrett be enrolled in an early intervention program as soon as possible. Faith scanned down the list of the programs provided to her by the professionals, realized she knew little about any of them, and decided to look them up on the Internet. One was described as a home-based applied behavior analysis program. Another was based on Relationship Development Intervention (Gutstein & Scheely, 2002), and a third employed Greenspan's Floortime (Greenspan, 2006) methodology. All of them described children's outcomes in reassuring language, but it was obvious that they were very different from one another. One required 30 hours per week of therapy and the others were two to three times per week for a couple of hours each. "Surely these differences must matter," she thought to herself. Faith logged on to a local Internet listserv for parents of children with autism to see what they were saying about the three programs. Faith soon discovered conflicting postings from parents. One parent wrote disparaging remarks about a program that another parent had said "saved" his child. Another parent described improvements in specific autism symptoms, like doubling of spontaneous speech over the past 3 months, while another referred to less tangible improvements, like reduced arousal and improved sensory modulation. Faith didn't know what to believe. She wondered how she could find out what intervention would really make the most difference for Garrett.

What Causes What?

Faith's question seemed straightforward: "If we enroll Garrett in Fizbee's Early Intervention Program, what change in his autism symptoms will likely occur, and over what time period?" This is a cause-and-effect question: If we do X (*cause:* intervention), will Y (*effect:* improved social and communication skills and fewer tantrums) follow? As simple as this seems, you may be surprised at how many people don't understand how to go about answering cause-and-effect questions.

In 1592, the founder of the modern scientific method, Francis Bacon, is claimed to have told the story of

> A grievous quarrel among the brethren (in a friary) over the number of teeth in the mouth of a horse. For thirteen days the disputation raged without ceasing. All the ancient books and chronicles were fetched out, and wonderful and ponderous erudition such as was never before heard of in this region was made manifest. At the beginning of the fourteenth day a youthful friar of goodly bearing . . . beseeched them to unbend in a manner coarse and unheard-of and to look in the open mouth of a horse and find answer to their questionings. At this, their dignity being grievously hurt, they waxed exceeding wroth; and, joining in a mighty uproar, they flew upon him and smote him, hip and thigh, and cast him out forthwith. (Mees, 1953, p. 383)

The notion of discovering what is and isn't the case by accurately observing nature has not always been popular. In some quarters it continues to be unpopular today.

The idea of using direct observation as a means of arriving at conclusions about what causes what has been around for a very long time. Prior to the 19th century, physicians treated people based on theories promulgated by theologians or philosophers, in the tradition of the horse's teeth example. Systematic observation of people's reactions to remedies played little role in deciding which treatments were most effective and therefore should continue to be used in the future.

The Scientific Method

The importance of scientific evidence as the basis for deciding upon treatments is not a new idea. With the emergence of early scientific medicine in the late 19th century, explicit rules emerged for deciding cause and effect. Instead of appealing to authorities such as philosophers or theologians when claiming that X caused Y, one was expected to present *empirical evidence* (i.e., information gained by means of systematic observation, experience, or experiment). Evidence of a causal link meant that one could demonstrate the relationships among events by watching, listening, or physically examining, or by using special instruments (like a microscope) to observe things too small to be seen by the naked eye. Hunches, opinions, or theories about whether X caused Y were no longer considered the basis for claiming a causal relationship. Today the scientific method consists of the collection of data through observing and experimentally manipulating factors thought to be related to outcomes, and the formulation and testing of hypotheses (Gauch, 2003).

Scientific Evidence Today

When we say we have scientific evidence, that means we have shown a reliable relation between a proposed cause and its effect, using agreed-upon observational procedures. The *scientific method* is the bedrock of medical and psychological science, but traditionally it hasn't been used in education. In testimony before the U.S. Senate and House committees on American education, Dr. A.K. Wigdor of the National Research Council remarked, "It is a striking fact that in the complex world of education—unlike defense, health care, or industrial production—personal experience and ideology are frequently relied on to make policy choices. In no other field is the research base so inadequate and so little used" (National Academies, 1999). But changes since that time have made the scientific method an increasingly important force in education, as well.

EVIDENCE-BASED MEDICINE

Among the foremost forces for change has been the emergence of *evidence-based medicine* (EBM). Prior to the 1990s, there was growing discontentment within clinical medicine regarding the lack of clear standards for evaluating treatments for various conditions. Almost anything could be called a treatment because there were no generally agreed-upon standards of medical evidence. In 1992, two prominent researchers in the United Kingdom presented a lecture that was published in a prestigious medical journal arguing for a standardized set of procedures for evaluating clinical research evidence (Lilford & Thornton, 1992). Subsequently, the Centre on Evidence-Based Medicine, the first of its kind, was established at Oxford University to study and promote EBM. That initial proposal grew into the more general concept of evidence-based *practice,* a movement that has spread throughout much of the world, and has now become the standard for evaluating evidence for many types of interventions in medicine, psychology, and education.

What Is Evidence-Based Medicine?

According to the Centre for Evidence-Based Medicine at Oxford University, "Evidence-based medicine is the conscientious, explicit and judicious use of current best evidence in making decisions about the care of individual patients" (Centre for Evidence Based Medicine, 2009). EBM requires finding the best evidence with which to answer a specific clinical question. It is important to weigh the *quality* of evidence concerning the risks and benefits of treatments. EBM recognizes that many aspects of medical care depend on individual factors such as quality-of-life judgments, which are only partially subject to scientific measurement. EBM, however, clarifies those parts of medical practice *that are in principle subject to scientific methods* and applies these methods to ensure the best prediction of outcomes in medical treatment. Evidence-based practice must also take into consideration the training and expertise of practitioners providing the services in question (Figure 5.1).

Evidence-Based Medicine in the United States

Within the United States, the U.S. Preventive Services Task Force of the Agency for Healthcare Research and Quality (2009) is an independent panel of experts that reviews the evidence of effectiveness and develops recommendations for clinical services. The task force adopted the standards of evidence developed by the Oxford Centre for Evidence Based Medicine in evaluating proposed treatments, with the strongest evidence for a treatment's effectiveness coming from Level I studies and the weakest evidence from Level III studies. Most autism treatment studies are Level II investigations,

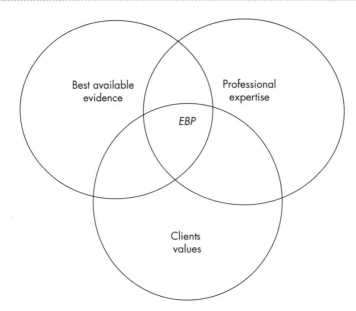

Figure 5.1. Diagram illustrating the elements making up evidence-based practice, which is shown by the intersection of best available evidence, professional expertise, and client or patient values.

providing intermediate-to-strong evidence, depending on the details of how the study was carried out.

- *Level I:* Evidence obtained from at least one randomized controlled trial (RCT) where participants are assigned to treatments by the flip of a coin and there is an untreated comparison group.

   Level II-1: Evidence obtained from controlled trials without assigning participants to groups randomly.

- *Level II-2:* Evidence obtained from studies in which, for every participant who receives the test treatment, another person who has similar characteristics will receive the control treatment or no treatment.

- *Level II-3:* Evidence obtained from studies in which a series of observations are made to establish a baseline, the intervention is implemented, and then more measurements are made to measure changes.

- *Level III:* Opinions of respected authorities, based on clinical experience, descriptive studies, or reports of expert committees.

Parents, Teachers, and Scientific Evidence

By now your head may be spinning. Why should parents, teachers, or other practitioners care about details of clinical research? For example, Faith, the mother whose dilemma we discussed in the previous section, is about to make a very important decision that may change the entire course of her son's life. Which type of early intervention is likely to produce the greatest long-term improvements in Garrett's functioning? Faith wants to know whether there is convincing evidence for the claim that one early intervention method yields better results than another for kids like Garrett. Answering that question requires evaluating the quality of the research that is the basis for that claim, which is why she needs a way of understanding the evidence.

Fortunately, Faith doesn't need to read the studies herself to evaluate the quality of the original research. She can rely on professionals who have reviewed all of the available published clinical or educational evidence and have concisely summarized it. They report how strong (or weak) the evidence really is. Those findings are published in articles in recognized scientific journals, within books, and are often reproduced in various parent web sites or print publications. Some are available online, such as the National Standards Project (http://www.nationalautismcenter.org/about/national.php).

Why Randomized Controlled Trials Are Often Difficult to Implement

Though RCTs—that is, studies in which children are assigned to a test treatment or a control or comparison treatment by the flip of a coin—may provide the strongest evidence, they are often very difficult to conduct when evaluating autism interventions. Few parents of a child with autism would agree to this procedure. Parents sense that every day counts for their child, and most consider it unacceptable for their child to be assigned to what may be a less effective intervention merely to find out whether the other intervention is more effective. Understandably, parents want their child to receive the most effective intervention immediately. Because of the overwhelming evidence that half of children with ASDs show dramatic improvement after receiving EIBI, professionals conducting intervention studies are faced with an ethical dilemma. Is it justifiable to provide half of a group of children with autism an intervention that is believed to be significantly less effective in order to answer the scientific question? If the jury were still out on that issue, one could rationalize such a study, but it isn't.

Studies involving random assignment of people to treatments are most readily conducted when the treatment is simple, such as taking a pill once a day for a week or a month, and when diagnosis of the condition being treated is clear, such as the height of the column of mercury when measuring high blood pressure. In evaluating treatment outcome in an RCT, a simple objective measure is most appealing. Complex measures that require teams of trained observers are less desirable in RCTs because they are more subject to errors of measurement. Different evaluators may conduct their observations in slightly different ways, yielding different results that actually may not be different.

In complex disorders such as ASDs, diagnosis can be thorny, and assignment of autism subtypes (e.g., Asperger syndrome, PDD-NOS, and Autistic Disorder) in equal proportions to intervention and control groups can be problematic. Not all treatment centers serve the same proportions of the three diagnostic subtypes. Some treatment centers may serve mainly children with Asperger syndrome and high functioning autism. Others may serve children with significant intellectual disability as well as autism. That means randomly selecting children from different types of centers will likely lead to an unbalanced assignment of children to interventions.

The longer an intervention must be in place (e.g., months or years versus weeks), the more difficult it becomes to ensure that the intervention has been carried out consistently across time. Not all interventions with the same name are implemented exactly the same way. Researchers attempt to solve this problem by providing an intervention manual that is to be followed by all practitioners at every treatment site.

Often the parents seeking diagnostic evaluations or intervention services for their children do so in a systematic (i.e., nonrandom) fashion. Parents from a given group within a community may gravitate toward a particular clinic because of word-of-mouth recommendations from other parents. Some parents seek clinics that support alternative medicine practices, while others do not. Randomly selecting participants from different clinics poses the problem that these different parental orientations may influence the way early interventions are implemented. Children and families enrolled in one clinic may not be representative of all children with ASDs. Limitations of randomized clinical trials are recognized in various areas of clinical medicine (McCulloch, Taylor, Sasako, Lovett, & Griffin, 2002).

Though RCTs have become the Holy Grail in many areas of clinical research, studies of groups selected based on matching characteristics may not only be more practical but may also provide better information, particularly with smaller sample sizes. A study conducted with children from a given school district or geographical area who receive an intervention being evaluated, compared with a "business as usual" intervention under the auspices of a single agency, is more likely to provide valid information than a multisite RCT at various sites around the country implemented by very different types of staff and somewhat different program approaches. Only with very large sample sizes does the latter approach make sense.

Evidence from Case-Controlled Studies

Most evidence regarding autism early intervention effectiveness comes from studies in which groups of children with similar characteristics received either early intervention or whatever services they would typically have received in their community (e.g., early childhood special education) *but are not randomly assigned to either service*. In this case, parents have selected their child's interventions. Some parents place a premium on having their child in a setting with other children their age, rather than receiving intensive one-to-one intervention services. In some cases, pairs of children are matched for similar characteristics—such as autism severity, intelligence scores, and language ability—at the beginning of the study. One child of each pair receives early intervention and the other receives the usual intervention provided in that program. When each pair of children has been enrolled in the study, intervention begins and additional pairs of participants are added until the number of children enrolled is sufficiently large for statistical analysis. Annually throughout intervention, independent, unbiased professionals evaluate each child's progress to determine whether there are emerging differences in outcomes. If the early intervention group achieves significantly more improvements in key measures than the other group using these methods, this is generally considered adequate evidence of effectiveness.

Some state agencies and insurance companies have denied reimbursement for EIBI services to preschool-age children with autism on the grounds that there are few true RCTs of such interventions. This denial may save money for state governments or insurance companies in the short run, but it is not a rational basis for reimbursing services and is more costly in the long term (Jacobson, Mulick, & Green, 1998). As we will discuss in Chapter 6, there have been more than 30 case-controlled and cohort studies, some with random assignment, that demonstrate the effectiveness of EIBI for young children with autism.

Anecdotal and Case Reports

Anecdotal reports from parents, no matter how sincere, cannot be considered scientific evidence. Nor can clinical case reports by a clinician who has treated a child and evaluated the outcome. A parent or a clinician has a vested interest in the outcome and cannot be considered an objective, unbiased observer. One of the most consistent and robust findings in clinical research is the *placebo effect* (Harrington, 1999). This refers to the fact that when a treatment is given to half of the participants in a clinical study and a sugar pill to the other half, a significant percentage of people receiving the sugar pill show improvements. Depending on the condition being treated, as many as 20% to 30% of people receiving the placebo report that they have improved. When a child is being treated for a condition such as autism or ADHD symptoms and their outcomes are being judged by a child's own parents, the placebo effect is often larger; in other words, parents of many of the kids receiving an ineffective intervention report their child has achieved substantial gains. Some of the most telling research has been with children with ADHD. Parents and teachers tend to evaluate children with ADHD more positively, and *they also behave more positively toward the children* when they believe the child has been administered stimulant medication. Parents and teachers also tend to attribute positive changes to medication even when the child is receiving a sugar pill (Waschbusch, Pelham, Waxmonsky, & Johnston, 2009).

Parents and the child's treating clinician hope and expect that the intervention being tried will reduce the child's symptoms and improve functioning. If they are aware of when the child is receiving the active intervention, then that may bias their evaluations of improvement. The same is true of behavioral or other nonmedication treatments. That is why anecdotal reports cannot be considered scientific evidence.

"If a parent sees improvement in their child, isn't the improvement real?" you might ask. No one doubts the parents' honesty or questions whether they believe they see improvement. The problems are the accuracy of their perceptions and their interpretation of what they have seen. There are many reasons why parents may believe their child's autism symptoms have improved, and accordingly, they attribute the alleged improvement to whatever intervention they have administered.

Consider the weather in England, which is famous for its fickle climate. When I lived in Cambridge, England many years ago, my British friends said, "If you don't like the weather, wait 15 minutes." Like the weather in England, daily and weekly fluctuations are the norm with autism, regardless of the intervention. On any given day or week a child's symptoms may seem improved or much worse. If the symptoms seem to be reduced (e.g., fewer tantrums), parents tend to attribute this improvement to whatever intervention is being employed at the time, especially if it is one in which they have an emotional investment. Such short-term fluctuations are seldom caused by a new intervention.

Improvements in core autism symptoms (communication and social skills and repetitive, restrictive behavior) are usually gradual over weeks and months and not usually apparent from day to day or week to week. Most children with autism receive multiple interventions at the same time, starting some and stopping others, sometimes at nearly the same time period. In the clinic with which I am affiliated, none of the children are receiving only EIBI. They all receive speech therapy, and most also receive occupational therapy. Some are on special diets, others receive supplements or have received chelating agents, and some have been taken by their parents to centers for hyperbaric oxygen treatment. That complicates the interpretion of changes in symptoms that may occur. For example, Nancy, the mother of a child with autism, recently told me that she had read an article in an autism publication that advocated a special diet. The author, an osteopathic physician, wrote that she had treated several children with the special diet, which she concluded had accounted for the children's improvements in autism symptoms. Nancy, who is an attorney and is a highly analytic thinker, reread the article more carefully. She noticed that in addition to the diet, all of the children also began receiving ABA therapy at about the same time. That was when Nancy began considering enrolling her child in an ABA early intervention program.

Some treatments, like stimulant medications for ADHD symptoms or some atypical antipsychotic medicines, may yield demonstrable improvements in attentiveness and reductions in impulsive, destructive behavior within days or a few weeks. But most interventions designed to improve a child's principal autism characteristics (i.e., social and communication skills) effect change much more gradually.

Evidence from Studies of Parts of Comprehensive Interventions

Few practitioners who work with children in schools or private homes have the resources to launch controlled studies of comprehensive interventions. But professionals working with service agencies or schools are often able to implement studies of parts of comprehensive interventions. Although such evidence doesn't prove the comprehensive interventions are effective, it lends credence to the possibility that the intervention strategy has merit, particularly if there are some larger scale studies as well.

Many clinical researchers have tested interventions to teach specific skills to children with autism and to overcome behavioral challenges. Several have combined those components into more comprehensive intervention strategies, though longitudinal group comparison studies of these treatments compared with untreated comparison groups have generally not been reported. For example, in their book *Pivotal Response Treatments for Autism,* Robert Koegel and Lynn Kern Koegel (2006) outlined intervention principles and illustrated their application to promote language and social skills, including initiations in school and during play dates. PRT is a naturalistic applied behavior analysis approach that incorporates developmental psychology concepts. Koegel and Koegel have published studies that have examined changes within each child's performance before and after components of PRT have been implemented. They have published numerous reports of individual components of PRT interventions indicating effectiveness of those methods in promoting specific skills and their generalization in natural settings. They have not, however, provided outcome data on comprehensive applications of all of their interventions in combination (i.e., comparing outcomes for groups of children receiving PRT versus a comparison intervention).

Vincent Carbone has developed an intervention approach called *Verbal Behavior* based on principles of ABA (Carbone, 2007). His clinical team developed methods for increasing requests and generalization of requests by children with autism by increasing the motivational value of the item being requested. In one study, the child's requests were brought under the control of their current motivational state (Sweeney-Kerwin, Carbone, O'Brien, Zecchin, & Janecky, 2007). In another, Carbone and colleagues used simultaneous presentation of a manual sign and associated spoken word, rather than teaching vocalization alone, yielding positive results (Carbone, Lewis, Sweeney-Kerwin, Dixon, Louden, & Quinn, 2006). Carbone and his colleagues have not conducted a comprehensive longitudinal study of outcomes for children receiving Verbal Behavior intervention compared with no intervention or "business as usual."

The lack of such comprehensive longitudinal study does not indicate that those methods are not effective. It means that data comparable to those of other ABA interventions have not been gathered.

SUMMARY

Parents and practitioners want information about the effectiveness of intervention options for their children and clients. Procedures have been developed that permit us to evaluate the quality of evidence regarding the effectiveness of various intervention options. The emergence of evidence-based practice has provided guidelines for assisting in such decision making. The most adequate evidence comes from controlled studies with random assignment of participants to interventions, or assigning matched pairs to intervention or a control group. Using these criteria, there is extensive evidence regarding the effectiveness of EIBI. Evidence for TEACCH and the Denver Early Start intervention models is encouraging. Numerous studies with components of other comprehensive interventions indicate that those components are effective, but evaluations of the entire intervention package remain to be done.

REFERENCES

Agency for Healthcare Research and Quality, U.S. Department of Health and Human Services. (2009). *U.S. Preventive Services Task Force.* Retrieved December 31, 2009, from http://www.ahrq.gov/clinic/uspstfix.htm

Carbone, V. (2007). *Carbone clinic.* Retrieved April 7, 2010, from http://www.drcarbone.net/

Carbone, V.J., Lewis, L., Sweeney-Kerwin, E.J., Dixon, J., Louden, R., & Quinn, S. (2006). A comparison of two approaches for teaching VB functions: Total communication vs. vocal alone. *Journal of Speech-Language Pathology and Applied Behavior Analysis, 1*(3), 181–192.

Centre for Evidence Based Medicine. (2009). *Centre for Evidence Based Medicine.* Retrieved December 31, 2009, from http://www.cebm.net/

Dickens, C. (1861/2008). *Great expectations.* Chapter XL(40). Project Gutenberg. [ebook #1400]. Release date August 20, 2008.

Gauch, Jr., H.G. (2003). *Scientific method in practice.* Cambridge, UK: Cambridge University Press.

Greenspan, S.I. (2006). *Engaging autism: Helping children relate, communicate and think with the DIR Floortime approach.* Cambridge, MA: Da Capo Lifelong Books.

Gutstein, S.E., & Sheely, R.K. (2002). *Relationship development intervention with young children: Social and emotional development activities for Asperger syndrome, autism, PDD and NLD.* London: Jessica Kingsley Publishers.

Harrington, A. (Ed.). (1999). *The placebo effect: An interdisciplinary exploration.* Cambridge, MA: Harvard University Press.

Jacobson, J.W., Mulick, J.A., & Green, G. (1998). Cost-benefit estimates for Early Intensive Behavioral Intervention for young children with autism. *Behavioral Interventions, 13,* 201–226.

Koegel, L.K., Koegel, R.L., Harrower, J.K., & Carter, C.M. (1999). Pivotal response intervention I: Overview of approach. *The Journal of the Association for Persons with Severe Handicaps, 24*(3), 174–185.

Koegel, R.L., & Koegel, L.K. (2006). *Pivotal Response Treatments for autism: Communication, social, and academic development.* Baltimore: Paul H. Brookes Publishing Co.

Lilford, R.J., & Thornton, J.D. (1992). Milroy Lecture 1992. *Journal of the Royal College of Physicians, 26*(4), 400–412.

McCulloch, P., Taylor, I., Sasako, M., Lovett, B., & Griffin, D. (2002). Randomised trials in surgery: problems and possible solutions. *British Medical Journal, 324,* 1448–1451.

Mees, C.E.K. (1953). Scientific thought and social reconstruction. *Electrical Engineering,* 383–384.

National Academies. (1999). *Testimony of Alexandra K. Wigdor on federal education research and evaluation efforts.* Retrieved December 31, 2009, from http://www7.nationalacademies.org/ocga/testimony/Federal_Education_Research_Evaluation_Efforts.asp

Sweeney-Kerwin, E.J., Carbone, V., O'Brien, L., Zecchin, G., & Janecky, N. (2007). Transferring control of the mand to the motivating operation in children with autism. *The Analysis of Verbal Behavior, 23,* 89–1102.

Waschbusch, D.A., Pelham, W.E.J., Waxmonsky, J., & Johnston, C. (2009). Are there placebo effects in the medication treatment of children with attention-deficit hyperactivity disorder? *Journal of Developmental and Behavioral Pediatrics, 30*(2), 158–168.

Early Intervention Dimensions

*"Before I built a wall I'd ask to know
What I was walling in or walling out,
And to whom I was like to give offense."*

—Robert Frost, *North of Boston* (1915)

Books and manuals on early intervention approaches for autism often define themselves as much by what their method *is not* as by what the method *is*. It is difficult for parents or practitioners to make sense of these conflicting statements about intervention policies and procedures. Most early intervention approaches have common features as well as obvious differences. Generally, little is said about common features.

Though differences among autism interventions are often emphasized in either-or terms, in practice they often exist on a continuum. Prizant and Wetherby (1998) wisely emphasized the continua along which intervention approaches vary and effectively summarized some of those dimensions. One example is the *degree of structure* involved. The UCLA Young Autism Project (Lovaas, 1987) and the TEACCH approach (Mesibov, Shea, & Schopler, 2004) are highly structured, whereas the Relationship Development Intervention (RDI; Gutstein & Sheely, 2002) and Floortime (Greenspan, 2006) methods are loosely structured. Pivotal Response Treatment (PRT; Koegel & Koegel, 2006) falls somewhere in between on the structure continuum. Though the UCLA Young Autism Model and TEACCH approach are both structured, their respective proponents often view them as being largely incompatible with one another on other grounds (Lovaas, Smith, & McEachin, 1989; Schopler, Short, & Mesibov, 1989).

Proponents tend to overemphasize and, at times, embellish differences among interventions. In this paragraph I italicize phrases that proponents of different intervention approaches have used to highlight what their approach *is not*, implying that other approaches exhibit those proscribed features. Stephen Gutstein and Rachel Sheely (2002, p. 23), creators of the RDI, wrote, "RDI is an invitational model. *You will not be coercing or bribing.*" This statement suggests that other early intervention approaches coerce and bribe. Mesibov, Shea, and Schopler (2004, p. 47) wrote of TEACCH, "Skills and behaviors are targeted for their functional utility for the individual's future, *rather than coming from lists of developmental sequences.*" In another place (p. 51), those authors wrote, "Unlike many ABA approaches, however, *TEACCH does not create structure by relying on repeated trials that begin with a prompt and are followed by material reinforcements.*" Thus, TEACCH distinguishes itself from other approaches that rely on developmental sequences (e.g., SCERTS) and repeated trials and material reinforcement (e.g., UCLA Young Autism Project). SCERTS training materials indicate that "the SCERTS Model

------

is not [italics in original] a curriculum focused solely on training skills *in a linear, lockstep manner"* (Prizant, Wetherby, Rubin, Laurent, & Rydell, 2005, p. 13), seemingly suggesting that other interventions teach skills in a lockstep fashion.

In his 1987 paper describing longitudinal outcomes for children with autism who received EIBI therapy, Ivar Lovaas distinguished his approach from psychodynamic treatments that had preceded him:

> Historically, psychodynamic theory has maintained a strong influence on research and treatment with autistic children, offering some hope for recovery through experiential manipulations. By the mid-1960s, an increasing number of studies reported that *psychodynamic practitioners were unable to deliver on that promise.* (Rimland, 1964)

Thus, Lovaas suggested that his ABA approach offers some hope for recovery, while psychodynamic approaches do not.

Sometimes, similar techniques are used by two early intervention models but are interpreted very differently within their respective theories. For example, both discrete trial ABA intervention and TEACCH employ extensive visual support strategies. Within ABA, visual supports are interpreted in terms of principles of discrimination learning, while within TEACCH, very similar methods are described as *visuospatial organization* (Mesibov, Shea, & Schopler, 2004). In this chapter, similarities as well as differences among early intervention approaches are discussed. Also, I examine some of the dimensions along which widely used early intervention approaches vary and consider which appear more relevant to child outcomes and which may not be as important, or else note where insufficient evidence exists one way or the other. The first section examines differences in developmental assumptions that underlie most of the disparities in approaches. Subsequent sections discuss resulting differences in intervention strategies and methods.

DEVELOPMENTAL ASSUMPTIONS

Cognitive Development

Disagreements regarding optimal early learning environments for children with autism begin with assumptions arising from the theoretical writings of Jean Piaget (1955) and Lev Vygotsky (1978), both of whom wrote about the development of neurotypical children. These theorists emphasized the importance of developmental appropriateness of materials available in the learning environment and viewed the teacher, parent, or therapist as a facilitator, not an instructor or therapist. Through exploring learning materials, these theorists assumed that a child moves from being undisciplined to self-disciplined, from disordered to ordered, and from distracted to focused.

Vygotsky (1978) maintained that a child naturally follows an adult's example and gradually develops the ability to do certain tasks without help or assistance. Vygotsky's most widely cited contribution is the *zone of proximal development* (ZPD), the range of tasks that are too difficult for the child to master alone but that can be learned with guidance and assistance of adults or more-skilled children. The lower limit of ZPD is the level of skill reached by the child working independently. The upper limit is the level of additional responsibility the child can accept with the assistance of an able instructor. The ZPD captures the child's cognitive skills that are in the process of developing and can be best accomplished with the assistance of a parent or other adult caregiver. *Scaffolding* is a concept closely related to the idea of ZPD. Scaffolding refers to changing the level of support. Over the course of a teaching session, an adult adjusts the amount of guidance to fit the child's current performance. This concept is similar to *shaping* and *prompt-fading* used in behavior analytic interventions.

In his extensive writings about children's learning, Piaget hypothesized that "authentic forms of intellectual exchange become possible" when the child has the freedom to project his or her own thoughts, consider the positions of others, and defend his or her own point of view (as cited in Muller, Carpendale, Budwig, & Sokol, 2008, p 183). Piaget's ideas were based on observing his own, presumably bright and verbally competent children. Piaget believed this led to "the reconstruction of knowledge," or favorable conditions for the emergence of constructive solutions to problems. He also argued that through a process of accommodation and assimilation, children construct new knowledge from their experiences. When a child *assimilates,* he or she incorporates the new experience into an existing framework without changing that framework. Although modern developmental psychologists tend to question the validity of Piaget's stage theory, it is generally agreed that contextualizing a child's experience makes sense, which is one of the reasons naturalistic or incidental learning strategies can be useful.

By contrast, young children with ASDs seldom learn from watching adult models, at least not until they explicitly have been taught to do so. Moreover, if children with ASDs are left to their own devices to learn through observing others, or through exploration of play or educational materials, they often lapse into repetitive, stereotyped behavior, such as rocking, flapping, and repeatedly banging or twirling play materials in nonfunctional ways. Many children on the autism spectrum do not spontaneously perceive toys or play materials as symbolically representing actual objects (e.g., cars, houses, people), except some highest functioning children. They must be explicitly taught component play skills that, when combined in a supportive context, yield useful functional activities. The strategy of multisensory experiential learning is seldom effective for young children with autism (Lord & McGee, 2001, p. 102).

SCERTS (Prizant, Wetherby, Rubin, Laurent, & Rydell, 2005) is one of the most complex, comprehensive approaches to autism early intervention. Though it emanates largely from a constructivist theoretical tradition, it incorporates concepts from behavior analysis learning theory approaches as well. The emphasis on child learning in natural environments and intrinsic motivation (i.e., avoiding consequences that are not indigenous to the context) is one of several features that distinguish the approach from discrete trial behavior analytic strategies. However, learning is more structured than recommended by other constructivist theorists.

ABA-based interventions are designed to provide children with autism with planned exposure to a range of developmentally appropriate stimuli, such as play materials and their partner's language and social cues. Specific skills appropriate to those stimuli are taught using principles of ABA, including stimulus supports and external rewards (e.g., social, preferred activities or material things). Most behavioral interventions are not discovery based like Montessori (1966) early intervention is.

Emotional Self-Regulation

A second underlying assumption of developmental approaches to early intervention is suppositions about *emotional self-regulation in autism*. Developmental psychologists have conducted extensive research on the processes by which typical infants and toddlers acquire the ability to regulate their feelings (Calkins & Fox, 2002). They have also studied emotional dysregulation among children with various forms (e.g., borderline personality disorder) of emotional disturbance (Kernberg & Michels, 2009). Emotional self-regulation involves the child's subjective experience of emotion, his or her thoughts in reaction to those feelings, physiological reactions within the body (e.g., heart rate, hormonal changes), and overt behavior (e.g., laughing, crying, facial expressions) related to emotion. Among neurotypical children, these processes depend on the child's developing capacities to discriminate between and interpret their own personal experiences. The process builds on emotional experiences from infancy. Gradually, these children begin to be more capable of managing their own feelings. By kindergarten, typical children often have the ability to anticipate, discuss, and use their awareness of their own and others' feelings in order to negotiate everyday social interactions. A typical 5-year-old might say, "I gave her my toy so she wouldn't feel bad," referring to his little sister (National Scientific Council on the Developing Child, 2004, p. 2). Several autism early intervention approaches attempt to directly promote emotional self-regulation, notably SCERTS, RDI, and Floortime.

The skills implicit in emotional self-regulation are among those that are typically absent or very limited in children with ASDs, such as distinguishing among one's own feelings. Their absence is one of the defining features of autism. There is little evidence from controlled studies that it is possible to directly change emotion self-regulation among children with autism, as proposed. I am reminded of the expression, "Get a hold of yourself!" which is intended to induce the listener to calm down, despite his or her emotional upheaval. If one could simply urge children with autism to "get a hold of" themselves and they would be able to do so, they would have many fewer difficulties. However, that rarely, if ever, works.

What little evidence exists suggests that changes in emotional self-regulation by children with autism come about by learning skills to gain control over dysregulating circumstances (e.g., being able to ask for help when facing a difficult task). Few behavioral interventions explicitly target regulation of internal feeling states as a goal, with the exception of PRT, which views it as a component of behavioral self-regulation (see Koegel, Koegel, Boettcher, Harrower, & Openden, 2006, pp. 247–248). Most behavior analytic-based interventions operate on the assumption that as children gain greater mastery of language and social skills and make cognitive gains, they have less reason for emotional distress. Their ability to emotionally self-regulate is thought to accompany those instrumental improvements in their daily relations with events and people around them. Adults who are trustworthy mediators of positive experiences and assist in relieving sources of negative feelings are vehicles for improved self-regulation. This assumption is similar to that in cognitive behavior therapy, namely that cognitive (e.g., language) and other behaviorally mediated skills gradually provide the framework within which feelings are interpreted and regulated (Thompson & Hollon, 2008).

HOW LEARNING OCCURS

Constructivist Developmental Approach to Early Learning

The manner in which early learning typically occurs differentiates intervention methods. As noted earlier, Floortime and RDI (to some degree) assume a child learns through exploration, intrinsic motivation, and coordinated emotional interactions with parents in the child's natural environment. Learning is not viewed as *goal-directed* activity—that is, it is not assumed that a child learns through attempting to achieve something and succeeding. Learning is seen as a *child-directed* process of discovering how the world works, including their emotional world. Developmental approaches to early intervention are rooted in constructivist theories of child development and learning that assume motivation to learn is an inherent characteristic of young children and is dependent on the child's confidence in his or her potential for learning. These feelings of competence are assumed to arise from mastery of problems in the past and are hypothesized to be more powerful than external acknowledgment or reinforcement (Prawat & Floden, 1994). Emphasis is placed on mastery motivation. External rewards—whether access to material things, preferred activities, or social recognition—are generally viewed as inappropriate, often postulated to undermine intrinsic motivation (Deci, Koestner, & Ryan, 1999; Lepper, Greene, & Nisbett, 1973). There is little evidence to support this assumption among children with autism and other developmental disabilities, but it is nonetheless a core assumption of developmental approaches to early intervention. (See Eisenberger and Cameron's 1996 review of this hypothesis with typical children in school settings.)

Behavior Analytic Approach to Early Learning

Bijou and Baer (1961) and Bijou and Baer (1965) first presented an organized theory of child development based on the premise that children learn mainly by associating what they do with the consequences of those actions, often in response to things said by parents, such as "Let's play Patty-cake" as a father holds up his hands, or "What does the doggy say?" According to this reasoning, the child learns that what they do or say works for them and is repeated, if something reliably happens as a result. The food reaches Libby's mouth, instead of falling off, if she holds her spoon just so and doesn't scoop too much on the spoon. And when Libby says, "Juice, please" and looks at her mother's eyes, Mom smiles at her and says, "Sure, Libby, here's juice" and hands her the sippy cup. Bijou and Baer (1961) emphasized that most social and language learning results from a child's interactions with his or her parents, siblings, peers, and, later, teachers, in which the child's actions become increasingly effective in producing the child's desired consequences. Behavior analytic early interventions operate from this premise.

In a sense, behavior analytic theory is more similar to psychodynamic theory than constructivist developmental theory. As in psychodynamic models, it is assumed that the child's behavior is goal-directed, based initially on basic biological drives but very soon making the transition to social motives. It is assumed that language learning mediates practical problem solving, reasoning, and organizing thoughts and feelings.

A child's success in making the world around him or her operate the way he or she wants serves to reward use of language or specific social skills such as looking at people when speaking to them. Each child gradually learns what works for her or him and achieves what she or he is striving for most efficiently. Making a verbal request for help is more efficient and requires less effort than crying for several minutes in order to obtain assistance. If the natural circumstances of the child's daily world do not provide opportunities to practice varied attempts at successfully communicating or socially engaging, which is typically the case for children on the autism spectrum, organized repetition of such experiences should be provided. This is what is attempted in ABA early intervention.

The notion that an ABA approach to learning in the daily environment involves artificially prompting a child (e.g., "Say, 'Ball'") and giving the child a piece of candy when he does so (Mesibov, Shea, & Schopler, 2004) caricatures the method's understanding of the way children's learning actually occurs in the natural environment. Although an ABA approach recognizes that learning may take place that way at times (e.g., when first starting early autism intervention), it is not usually the way learning occurs in practice during a child's daily experience. Following are some typical situations where learning occurs, based upon behavior analytic assumptions:

·   When 3-year-old Polly wants to play and looks up at her Dad and says, "Horsey?" her father rewards the child's utterance by hoisting Polly on his shoulders. He says, "Okay, let's play Horsey" as he makes whinnying sounds and marches about the living room giving Polly a bumpy horseback ride. If Polly's stated request isn't sufficiently clear, Dad doesn't understand what Polly says, so her inarticulate utterance is unsuccessful (i.e., is not reinforced). Eventually Polly learns to say, "Horsey" more clearly, because it is more effective in communicating with her father and leads to the consequence she wants. Dad doesn't plan to artificially reinforce Polly's utterance, which is just the way the world works.

·   Adam holds up a felt-tip pen drawing he just completed to show his mother. She says, "That's a terrific doggy! What nice ears she has," remarking about the dog's long purple ears. Mother's presence was a cue (technically called a *discriminative stimulus*) to Adam to show her his drawing, and her comments reinforced both drawing the picture and showing her his artwork (lack of showing is a common autism deficit).

·   During intensive early behavior therapy taking place on a blanket in a family's backyard, Amy, a behavior therapist, is discussing the color of the sky with Duante. Amy says, "Look!" and points at birds flying in the sky. Duante looks up and then notices another object moving more rapidly across the sky, and the therapist says, "What is that?" Duante watches for a moment and says, "Airplane." "Wow, that's right, it's an airplane," Amy answers. "Is anything else in the sky?" Duante looks around for another few seconds and says, "Sun and clouds." "There are lots of things in the sky today," Amy replies. This is the way learning usually occurs in the natural environment, viewed within the framework of behavior analytic concepts and, during therapy, through simulation of the natural environment.

Adult-Directed versus Child-Directed Learning

Maria Montessori (1966) suggested that children learn best when they follow their own interests. This is a bedrock assumption of most developmental approaches and makes sense, at least up to a point. A child is likely to be more motivated by a red toy car that he or she can push across the floor than by a red square painted on a piece of paper. Within PRT, therapists are encouraged to identify what the child is interested in during an initial assessment and use those things or activities as motivators (Koegel, Openden, Freeden, & Koegel, 2006). Among children with more cognitive limitations and who have more severe autism symptoms, a child's interests may be extremely narrow and dysfunctional, such as twirling pieces of string in circles, flipping light switches on and off, or mouthing objects. The child may also have very limited ability to attend to a task for more than a few seconds at a time. If such a child is allowed to do so, he or she may devote a large proportion of his or her time to such repetitive nonfunctional stereotypical activities and resist redirection. Over the course of a child-determined learning or therapy session (i.e., following the child's lead), such a child would have very few opportunities to learn more adaptive skills.

To address this problem, therapists or teachers employing a DTI approach determine most of the content of activities in which a child is engaged. They begin by teaching the child to "come sit" (pointing to a chair at a child-sized table) as a means of focusing the child's attention. They then model and reinforce the child's simple motor imitation activities, such as clapping hands. Each sequence of activities occurs for a very short period in the beginning (e.g., 5–10 minutes), followed by a reinforcing activity (e.g., tickles) or edible treat (e.g., small piece of fruit).

In RDI, the adult is called a coach, facilitator, and friend, not a teacher or therapist. To structure the child's experiences, 138 activities are provided to promote 12 stages of relationship skills (Gutstein & Sheely, 2002, p. 25). One such activity, "Follow My Eyes to the Prize," teaches the child to find a hidden object by following the adult's eye gaze. This procedure is adult-directed within an overall child-led therapy strategy; it is similar to one we use at the Minnesota Early Autism Project with higher functioning children on the autism spectrum to teach the child to attend to eye gaze and facial expression. In PRT, the child selects the stimulus by touching it or pointing to it and the clinician says the name of the item (e.g., "car"). The child and clinician play with the item. Then the child attempts to respond by naming the item, which is loosely reinforced using natural consequences (e.g., opportunity to play with the item; Koegel, Openden, et al., 2006). Thus, the adult structures the situation but responds flexibly to opportunities provided by the child's behavior. On the continuum between following the child's lead and adult-directed activities, PRT is somewhere in the middle.

Individual versus Group Learning

Early intervention services occur in two types of settings: 1) one-to-one interaction between a trained teacher, therapist, or parent and the child with autism; or 2) intervention with the child with autism in a congregate setting, such as an early childhood special education classroom.

Among one-to-one interaction services, ZERO-TO-THREE programs operated by state agencies often contract with public schools to provide home-based services in which teachers, speech therapists, or occupational therapists come into the child's home a few hours per week. Parents are encouraged to observe and carry out the same procedure on their own. Although this is a good start, this level of intervention is generally insufficient to meet the needs of most children with autism. EIBI services also are often home-based and involve a team of therapists working in shifts with the child, 25–35 hours per week, one to one.

The second type of setting is in a school- or center-based program. Parents want their son or daughter with autism to have fun playing with other children and learning to socialize. As a result, they often enroll their 4-year-olds with autism in a special education preschool, often 3 half-days per week. This may be helpful for higher functioning children with strong social interests, especially if they have had prior intensive home-based therapy. However, some children with ASDs have no interest in other children and may actively avoid them. Being in a classroom of noisy children may seem unpleasant and distressful to many children on the autism spectrum. Often they would prefer being at home with Mom or Dad, a sibling, and their family dog. Few children with ASDs, even those with Asperger syndrome or PDD-NOS, have any idea how to interact with their peers. They may observe other children playing and then retreat to play with a toy in isolation or stare out the window. Some children with whom we have worked are eager to try to join in other children's play but do so ineptly and are rebuffed. After several attempts, they often give up. In order for classroom participation to be *a meaningful social experience,* most children with autism must be taught prerequisite social and communication skills.

Some children participate in specialized private schools for children with autism or, sometimes, with mixed disabilities. Typically, in those settings, most instruction is one to one or one to two but is often interspersed with group activities—such as physical education, art, music, or lunch—with peers with disabilities. Because the staff ratios are higher and staff have specialized autism training, it may be more likely children will have positive social experiences in these settings than in a typical larger public school classroom, especially one led by a general education teacher. Successful participation in a school setting depends on the student-to-staff ratio, teacher training and experience, and the curriculum.

Children participating in RDI have ample time for taking part in preschool because typically the Relationship Development Intervention professional coach only works with the child 4 to 8 hours per week, one to one and with parents. Similarly, PRT is often conducted several hours weekly in collaboration with parents and teacher when children are enrolled in school. In both cases (RDI and PRT), parents and teachers are encouraged to carry out therapy on their own. Children participating in TEACCH usually receive service in school, but more often when they are in elementary school. Children taking part in Floortime receive similar intensity of services from trained consultants at home, but parents are told that for more severe and challenging problems, eight to ten parent-administered 20- to 30-minute Floortime sessions every day is optimal. If parents actually carry out Floortime activities with this intensity, it would be difficult for the child to participate in preschool in addition. However, Floortime recommends regular peer playdates and sibling socialization activities (Greenspan, 2004), which compensates.

Many discrete trial ABA programs encourage parents to make their children available for a minimum of 25–35 hours per week of one-to-one therapy, which together with speech and any other therapies would generally preclude participation in preschool. This can be a source of conflict with school districts, which typically contend that they are able to provide appropriate services to children with autism.

When children are higher functioning and have clear social interest, we encourage parents to enroll their 4- to 5-year-old youngsters with autism in preschool approximately 6 to 9 hours per week, a time period that usually includes speech therapy. We work with the child to develop peer "joining in" and other social and communication skills to make their time in school more enjoyable, and consult with classroom teachers on which skills would be helpful for the child to be more successful at school.

Participation in General Education

The decision to enroll a child in a classroom for neurotypical students versus a program for children with disabilities can be difficult. Children of ages 3 or 4 with autism can seldom profit from participating in a general education preschool program without supplementary supports, including prerequisite training and ongoing paraprofessional support in consultation with the school's autism specialist. Once they have had 2 or more years of intensive intervention, about half of them can profit from a school setting with minimal supports.

Special Education Placement

Placing a child in a classroom where most of the children have significant disabilities can also have disadvantages. Such a segregated setting provides few positive models. Moreover, if most of the other students have an ASD, they will likely be relatively unresponsive to a new student in their midst, which means social overtures will not be re-turned and are less likely to lead to friendships. If a child has lower cognitive functioning and more severe autism symptoms, such a setting may be appropriate, depending on skills of the instructional staff and the curriculum.

High versus Low Intensity

There is ample evidence that increases in language, social skills, and adaptive skills are directly related to therapy intensity (hours per week of service; Eikeseth, Smith, Jahr, & Eldevik, 2007; Eldevik, Eikeseth, Jahr, & Smith, 2006). The more hours of intervention services a child receives, the greater will be the cognitive, social, and language improvements. But Warren, Fey, and Yoder (2007) pointed out that there is more to therapy intensity than number of hours a therapist or teacher is with a child. For example, many of us of have seen situations in which an interventionist repeatedly uses an instructional or therapy procedure that produces little or no improvement in a child's functioning. That shouldn't happen, but it does. Further repetitions of such an ineffective procedure don't constitute greater therapy intensity. *Intensity* refers to amount of *effective* service.

Existing evidence indicates that *on average, more intervention is better,* at least up to a point. Low intensity of ABA therapy—15 hours per week, for example—may not be sufficient to make major symptom improvements over the first 1–2 years of therapy (Smith, Groen, & Wynn, 2000).

There is a great range of service intensity among autism early interventions. Proponents of DTI usually argue for a minimum of 30–35 hours of one-to-one therapy with a trained person. RDI coaches work with a child and parents two to three times per week for several hours on each occasion. Parents are encouraged to use the same methods on their own the rest of the time. PRT (Koegel, Openden, et al., 2006) and Floortime (Greenspan & Wieder, 2009, p. 186) both recognize the importance of therapy intensity but assume parents are willing and able to make up the remaining hours needed to make major gains. TEACCH is typically conducted in schools on half-days with kindergarten children or for 6 hours per day with elementary school children. Similarly, SCERTS is viewed primarily as a form of intervention to be carried out in schools by speech therapists and special education teachers, though it can also be done at home. (SCERTS is a very complex intervention system. Most parents would require considerable support to be able to employ the suggested methods on their own.) Professional contact time with the child is limited by typical ratios in schools, again with the assumption that other school personnel will employ similar procedures on their own.

Reliance on Parents and Teachers to Conduct Independent Interventions

Research on adherence (Moore & Symons, 2009) to recommended treatments is not encouraging, raising doubts about the assumption that parents or teachers will independently carry out recommended therapy methods with sufficient consistency or intensity. There are many other competing demands, making it difficult for parents and teachers to do so. Studies of adherence to even simple treatments, like taking pills or using inhalers once or several times daily, have found low levels of adherence to recommended treatments. For example, Moore and Symons (2009) summarized adherence to medical treatments. They found that in treating Type 1 diabetes and asthma, there is between 30% and 98% nonadherence to drug and related therapies, even though untreated episodes could be potentially fatal. Only 50%–70% of psychiatric patients adhere to medication regimens, and 40% to 60% of those people terminate treatment early. Bear in mind that these treatments only require a few minutes per day and little disruption of normal daily routine. It seems unlikely that the far more complex and demanding behavioral/psychological or educational treatments involved in autism early intervention would be implemented by parents and teachers with greater consistency or fidelity. It is possible that a lower level of adherence may be capable of producing child improvements, but it seems unlikely that such improvements would be comparable to those resulting from 25 to 30 hours per week of one-to-one therapy. Relying on parents or teachers to carry out interventions almost entirely on their own will likely yield lower intensity levels than those implemented by trained staff members in collaboration with parents.

I would like to be very clear that low levels of parental adherence do not reflect lack of parental commitment or desire to support their children's development. It may be unrealistic to ask parents to adopt intervention methods that may seem somewhat alien to them and engage in activities that compete with many other demands on their time, such as other child care, managing the household, and attending to extended family commitments (Grindle, Kovshoff, Hastings, & Remington, 2009). It is not safe to assume that somehow parents will find the time to insert substantial therapy activities within their daily routines.

Learning within Natural Daily Routines versus Controlled Therapy or Learning Situations

Home-based DTI is often conducted at a child-sized table in a room set aside specifically for therapy. Therapy may initially occur in a family room, recreation room, or a spare bedroom. The goal is to minimize distractions and help the child learn that when she or he is seated at the table with a therapist, she or he is expected to participate in adult-directed activities. Early in therapy, siblings or ongoing activities in the home are excluded from the therapy area to avoid distractions. With time, parents and siblings become involved in therapy activities; later, peers are included as well. Therapy activities are based on initial and subsequent assessments of skill deficits that impede the child's typical functioning, mainly communication and social skills but also including play and cognitive skills. Instruments such as the Assessment of Basic Language and Learning Skills-Revised (Partington, 2007) or the Verbal Behavior Milestones Assessment and Placement Program (Sundberg, 2008) evaluate adequacy of specific skills in important domains that become the targets of teaching or therapy. These instruments provide examples of suggested activities for each item on each scale.

Floortime is conducted at home and may include parents and siblings. Instead of using a table as the location where therapy activities occur, the therapist sits on the floor with the child and conducts therapy activities there. Hence, behavior analysis's DTI's Tabletime is replaced by Greenspan's Floortime. Developmental assessments of attention, sensorimotor, gestures, problem solving, and symbolic play are used as a basis for planning intervention (Greenspan, deGangi, & Wieder, 2001). The assessment does not prescribe activities to promote specific skills; rather, it suggests categories of developmental competence as beginning points for intervention (e.g., Child Scale, item 10: "Evidences a relaxed sense of security and/or comfort when near caregiver. If child is active and moves away from caregiver, he references her from across space and shows relaxed security in distal space.") Loosely structured activities are employed based on the child's interests and his or her beginning developmental levels according to the assessment. Activities are designed to encourage the child's initiative, purposeful behavior, engagement, lengthening mutual attention, and developing symbolic capacities through pretend play and conversations, while following the child's lead. These activities are not spontaneous in the sense that a child moves haphazardly from one activity to another; the therapist (or parent) creates the context for and guides the activity (e.g., hiding a toy under sand in a sandbox).

PRT employs normal daily activities at home and typical preschool activities at school, with modifications for the special needs of children with autism (Koegel, Openden, Freeden, & Koegel, 2002, pp. 15–20). Modified discrete trial procedures are embedded within typical daily routines at home and school, employing materials and activities indigenous to those settings. Emphasis is placed on promoting language by providing highly motivating toys and other materials distributed throughout the natural environment. A common procedure is to place desired items out of reach so that the child will have to use gestures and/or speech to gain access to them. Coordination of procedures developed at home with those being implemented at school is an important emphasis of this approach. PRT piggybacks onto the preschool curriculum and does not provide the same kind of independent, comprehensive interventions as those employed in SCERTS or DTI, which grow out of detailed assessments of developmental skills, or the curriculum-based assessments indicated previously.

Parents as Primary Therapists, Cotherapists, or Service Coordinators

The degree and type of parent involvement varies greatly from family to family. Participation often depends on where parents are in the process of accepting their child's disability. Parents who are struggling to accept their child's diagnosis and who are very actively pursuing a wide array of alternative treatments in the hope that one will lead to their child's recovery usually find it difficult to participate in therapy. Each session they work with their child is a reminder of their child's very significant deficits and how different he or she is from typically developing sisters or brothers or the neighbor child. Incremental enhancement of their child's functioning may be very frustrating to some parents, because their goal may be to cure their child's autism, not make stepwise progress toward more typical functioning.

In Relationship Development Intervention, Floortime, and PRT, it is assumed that most of the therapy will be implemented by the child's parents. Procedures are described and demonstrated by trained professionals, who provide educational and emotional support, at which point parents are expected to take over. In DTI the opposite is usually the case (i.e., most of the therapy is provided by trained practitioners, with parents employing some of the same procedures when therapists are not present); parents are involved in planning, setting goals, and evaluating progress, but seldom take the lead in conducting therapy.

I have worked with some especially motivated and engaged parents who eagerly adapt therapy procedures to novel situations when therapists aren't present. For example, Jesi's parents took her by airplane to visit their family in another state. Jesi had been taught by therapy staff to wear earphones and listen to preferred music when she was in noisy settings that she found disturbing, such as when her mom was vacuuming the rug. Waiting for their flight at the airport was another one of those noisy settings, with public address announcements blaring loudly, carts making beeping sounds, and the roar of jet engines. Jesi's mom dug through her carry-on bag and found Jesi's earphones and CD player. Jesi put on the earphones, punched the button on the CD player, and began listening to one of her favorite Motown hits, closing her eyes and swinging her head from side to side with the rhythm of the music. Jesi's world had suddenly become manageable. Jesi's parents do very well participating in a type of early intervention therapy that involves more independent parent involvement (for more about Jesi, see Chapter 7).

Other parents prefer to observe therapy procedures and understand their rationale, but minimally employ therapy methods on their own. They may have a college education and may be intensely interested in the latest research on autism. Many such parents attend workshops and read books on autism on their own. They often ask insightful questions. Mom drives her child to speech and occupational therapy and to their three-morning-a-week early childhood special education classes and oversees numerous other professional appointments. In my experience, such parents are often diligent in attending therapy team meetings and making suggestions, participating in parent–teacher conferences at school, and negotiating with funding agencies for reimbursement for their child's services. They are parents who thrive in the role of their child's service coordinator but shy away from being their child's main hands-on therapists. They feel they are doing what they can do best for their child.

Floortime, RDI or PRT therapy may be more appealing to some parents because the therapy process often feels familiar to them and makes minimal demands of them (other than the two or three sessions per week). Though parents are recommended by these approaches to conduct eight to ten 20-to-30 minute therapy sessions daily on their own (Greenspan & Wieder, 2009), in practice they can pick and choose when they actually use those same methods. In some cases, it may be unlikely that they devote the prescribed time.

DTI therapy approaches may be seen by some parents as freeing them from the responsibility for carrying most of the therapy. Parents whose children are receiving 30 to 35 hours per week of DTI are making significant sacrifices of their family life and often making financial commitments as well (Grindle, Kovshoff, Hastings, & Remington, 2009). There is no question that they are dedicated to doing what they think is best for their child, but for some parents it is extremely difficult to play a leading role in the performance that is their child's therapeutic life (Remington et al., 2007).

One of the more common parent involvement scenarios begins with Mom and Dad becoming actively involved in overcoming their child's challenging behavior, such as meltdowns. For example, Jack and Tammy eagerly sought help in overcoming Christopher's tantrums and judiciously carried out recommended procedures for overcoming them. The strategy involved identifying situations that predisposed Christopher to an outburst and teaching something else he could do in those circumstances that served a similar purpose, such as delaying completion of a task for a few minutes. With persistence, Tammy and Jack experienced success and were justifiably pleased with their own achievement as Christopher's meltdowns dwindled.

Then an unexpected benefit of their success occurred. They began to employ other recommended procedures that fit in well with their daily routines, such as at mealtimes, bathing, and getting ready for bed. For example, they effectively carried out recommended mealtime conversation procedures that incorporated Christopher, because family members are all at the dinner table anyway. The recommended procedures were simple and very doable. Over several weeks, mealtimes were transformed from a night-mare, with screaming and throwing food, into a pleasant daily family social ritual. Tammy and Jack continued to find it difficult to insert additional therapy activities into their daily schedules that took them outside of their normal routines. Parents gen-erally do what they can do, which is as it should be. Parents should be parents, not ther-apists. Having unrealistic expectations of parents isn't helpful.

CONCLUSIONS

Autism and its treatment has become the latest battlefield among psychology's warring factions, which is not of benefit to children with autism and their families. Descendents of John B. Watson's behaviorism (1913) and B.F. Skinner's behavior analy-sis (1938, 1953) are lined up on one side, and followers of the constructivist develop-mental theorists descended from Jean Piaget (1955) and Lev Vygotsky (1978), and psychodynamic theorists Erik Erikson (1968) and John Bowlby (1969), are on the other. *Behaviorism* is an empirical research tradition with emphasis on measurement, and *con-structivism* is a theoretical clinical tradition, which is often more qualitative. People in the behavioral tradition are more focused on objective outcomes, and those in the lat-ter camp seek a theoretical explanation consistent with their concept of human nature. What solid empirical evidence we have concerning autism early intervention is largely from the former rather than the latter. None of this theoretical quarreling is helpful.

Figure 6.1 shows dimensions along which widely disseminated and/or replicated early intervention therapies are similar and different. For example, both DTI and TEACCH are mostly adult directed, high intensity, and the parent's role is that of a team member and not the primary therapist. They differ, however, on the source of child motivation, with DTI using extrinsic rewards and TEACCH relying more on mas-tery motivation. It is noteworthy that PRT and Blended Behavioral Interventions fall closer to the midpoint on these various dimensions, incorporating elements of both adult and child-directed, some high intensity but also lower intensity intervention and both individual and group intervention. There are, of course, many other site-specific programs that have done important work as well (see Lord & McGee, 2001), but those programs have not been widely disseminated among other sites. Though proponents of various approaches often emphasize dichotomous theoretical differences, in prac-tice, as therapies are actually implemented, there are often similarities.

We do not need to wait for the theoretical disagreements about the nature of human nature to be settled in order to provide more adequate early intervention ser-vices for the wide range of young children with autism. Chapters 9 and 10 explore blended interventions that incorporate components of developmentally based strate-gies within a behavior analytic approach that have proven effective and make sense.

Dimensions	100%	75%/25%	50%/50%	25%/75%	100%		Dimensions
Adult-directed	DTI	TEACCH	PRT, SCERTS, Blended	RDI	Floortime	Incidental, follow child's lead	Adult- or child-directed
High	DTI	Blended, TEACCH	SCERTS, PRT	RDI	Floortime	Low	Intensity*
Extrinsic	DTI	Blended	PRT, TEACCH	SCERTS, RDI	Floortime	Intrinsic, mastery	Motivation
One-to-one	RDI, DTI, Floortime		PRT, Blended	SCERTS	Floortime	Group	Individual or group learning
Autism only	TEACCH, DTI	RDI, Floortime	Blended	SCERTS	TEACCH	Autism typical	Autism only or integrated
Secondary to skills	DTI, TEACCH	Blended	PRT		RDI, SCERTS, Floortime	Primary focus	Emotional self-regulation
Team member	DTI, TEACCH		SCERTS, Blended	PRT	RDI, Floortime	Primary therapist	Parent role

Figure 6.1. Dimensions along which common autism early interventions can be compared and contrasted. Columns 3 to 7 indicate relative balance (expressed as percentages) of the extremes of each dimension associated with various common autism interventions. Titles of dimensions are shown in the first column and the contrasting opposites are shown in the second and eighth (far right) column. It is noteworthy that there are similarities among some dimensions for interventions that have very different theoretical foundations, whereas others differ considerably among dimensions.
(Key: DTI, Discrete Trial Intervention; RDI, Relationship Development Intervention; SCERTS=Social Communication, Emotional Regulation and Transactional Support; TEACCH=Treatment and Education of Autistic and Communication-Related Handicapped Children. Percentage headings: 100%, all intervention on a given dimension is at one end of the continuum; 75%/25%, approximately three quarters of the intervention on that dimension is at one end of the continuum and one quarter at the other end; 25%/75%, approximately one quarter of the intervention is at one end of the continuum and three quarters at the other end; 50%/50%, approximately equal involvement of both ends of the continuum.)
 * **Intensity** refers to the total number of hours per week of effective intervention engagement. High intensity usually refers to 25+ hours per week, low intensity refers to 12 or fewer hours per week, intermediate intensity refers to 13–24 hours per week.

REFERENCES

Bijou, S.W., & Baer, D.M. (1961). *Child development* (vol. 1). New York: Appleton Century Crofts.

Bijou, S.W., & Baer, D.M. (1965). *Child development* (vol. 2). New York: Appleton-Century-Crofts.

Bowlby, J. (1969). *Attachment* (vol. 1). New York: Basic Books.

Calkins, S.D., & Fox, N.A. (2002). Self-regulatory processes in early personality development: A multilevel approach to the study of childhood social withdrawal and aggression. *Developmental Psychopathology, 14*(3), 477–498.

Carbone, V. (2007). *Carbone clinic.* Retrieved April 7, 2010, from http://www.drcarbone.net/

Carbone, V.J., Lewis, L., Sweeney-Kerwin, E.J., Dixon, J., Louden, R., & Quinn, S. (2006). A comparison of two approaches for teaching VB functions: Total communication vs. vocal alone. *Journal of Speech-Language Pathology and Applied Behavior Analysis, 1*(3), 181–192.

Deci, E.L., Koestner, R., & Ryan, R.M. (1999). A meta-analytic review of experiments examining the effects of extrinsic rewards on intrinsic motivation. *Psychological Bulletin, 125*(6), 627–668; discussion 692–700.

Eikeseth, S., Smith, T., Jahr, E., & Eldevik, S. (2007). Outcome for children with autism who began intensive behavioral treatment between ages 4 and 7: A comparison controlled study. *Behavior Modification, 31*(3), 264–278.

Eisenberger, R., & Cameron, J. (1996). Detrimental effects of reward: Reality or myth? *American Psychologist, 51,* 1153–1166.

Eldevik, S., Eikeseth, S., Jahr, E., & Smith, T. (2006). Effects of low-intensity behavioral treatment for children with autism and mental retardation. *Journal of Autism and Developmental Disorders, 36*(2), 211–224.

Erikson, E.H. (1968). *Identity: Youth and crisis.* New York: W.W. Norton & Company.

Frost, R. (1915). *North of Boston* [Electronic version]. Retrieved January 1, 2010, from http://www.gutenberg.org/catalog/world/readfile?fk_files=1074378

Greenspan, S. (2004). Best understanding of autism spectrum disorders. Web Based radio show. May 13, 2004. Retrieved November 3, 2010, from http://www.icdl.com/distance/webRadio/documents/5-13-04.pdf

Greenspan, S.I. (2006). *Engaging autism: Helping children relate, communicate and think with the DIR Floortime approach.* New York: Da CapoBooks.

Greenspan, S.I., deGangi, G., & Wieder, S. (2001). *The functional emotional assessment scale (FEAS) for infancy and early childhood: Clinical and research applications.* Bethesda, MD: Interdisciplinary Council on Developmental and Learning Disorders.

Greenspan, S.I., & Wieder, S. (2009). *Engaging autism: Helping children relate, communicate and think with the DIR Floortime approach.* New York: Da Capo Books.

Grindle, C.F., Kovshoff, H., Hastings, R.P., & Remington, B. (2009). Parents' experiences of home-based applied behavior analysis programs for young children with autism. *Journal of Autism and Developmental Disorders, 39*(1), 42–56.

Gutstein, S.E., & Sheely, R.K. (2002). *Relationship development intervention with young children: Social and emotional development activities for Asperger syndrome, autism, PDD and NLD.* London: Jessica Kingsley Publishers.

Kernberg, O.F., & Michels, R. (2009). Borderline personality disorder. *American Journal of Psychiatry, 166*(5), 505–508.

Koegel, L.K., Koegel, R.L., Boettcher, M.A., Harrower, J., & Openden, D. (2006). Combining functional assessment and self-management procedures to rapidly reduce disruptive behaviors. In R.L. Koegel & L.K. Koegel (Eds.), *Pivotal Response Treatments for autism: Communication, social, and academic development* (pp. 247–248). Baltimore: Paul H. Brookes Publishing.

Koegel, R.L., & Koegel, L.K. (2006). *Pivotal Response Treatments for autism: Communication, social, and academic development.* Baltimore: Paul H. Brookes Publishing Co.

Koegel, R.L., Openden, D.F., Freeden, R.M., & Koegel, L.K. (2006). The basics of pivotal response treatment. In R.L. Koegel & L.K. Koegel (Eds.), *Pivotal response treatments for autism* (p. 11). Baltimore: Paul H. Brookes Publishing Company.

Lepper, M.R., & Greene, D. (1978). *The hidden costs of reward: New perspectives on the psychology of human motivation.* Mahwah, NJ: Lawrence Erlbaum Associates.

Lepper, M.R., Greene, D., & Nisbett, R.E. (1973). Undermining children's intrinsic interest with extrinsic rewards: A test of the "overjustification" hypothesis. *Journal of Personality and Social Psychology, 28,* 129–137.

Lord, C.E., & McGee, J. (2001). *Educating children with autism.* Committee on Behavioral Sciences, National Research Council. Washington, DC: National Academies Press.

Lovaas, O.I. (1987). Behavioral treatment and normal educational and intellectual functioning in young autistic children. *Journal of Consulting and Clinical Psychology, 55*(1), 3–9.

Lovaas, O.I., Smith, T., & McEachin, J.J. (1989). Clarifying comments on the young autism study: Reply to Schopler, Short, and Mesibov. *Journal of Consulting and Clinical Psychology, 57*(1), 165–167.

Mesibov, G.B., Shea, V., & Schopler, E. (2004). *The TEACCH approach to autism spectrum disorders (issues in clinical child psychology).* New York: Springer.

Montessori, M. (1966). *The secret of childhood.* Notre Dame, IN: Fides Publishers.

Moore, T.R., & Symons, F.J. (2009). Adherence to behavioral and medical treatment recommendations by parents of children with autism spectrum disorders. *Journal of Autism and Developmental Disorders, 39*(8), 1173–1184.

Mosby. (2009). *Mosby's Medical Dictionary* (8th ed., p. 2056). New York: Elsevier.

Muller, U., Carpendale, J.I.M., Budwig, N., & Sokol, B. (2008) Social life and social knowledge: Toward a process account of development. Page 183. Mahwah, NJ: Lawrence Erlbaum Associates.

National Scientific Council on the Developing Child. (2004). *Children's emotional development is built into the architecture of their brains: Working paper no. 2.* Retrieved January 2, 2010, from http://www.developingchild.harvard.edu

Partington, J. (2007). ABLLS-R: The assessment of basic language and learning skills-revised. Walnut Creek, CA: The Behavior Analysts, Inc.

Piaget, J. (1955). *Construction of reality in the child* (M. Cook, Trans.). Routledge and Kegan Paul.

Prawat, R.S., & Floden, R.W. (1994). Philosophical perspectives on constructivist views of learning. *Educational Psychology, 29,* 37–48.

Prizant, B.M., & Wetherby, A.M. (1998). Understanding the continuum of discrete-trial traditional behavioral to social-pragmatic developmental approaches in communication enhancement for young children with autism/PDD. *Seminars in Speech and Language, 19*(4), 329–52.

Prizant, B.M., Wetherby, A.M., Rubin, E.M.S., Laurent, A.C., & Rydell, P.J. (2005). *The SCERTS model: A comprehensive educational approach for children with autism spectrum disorders* (vols. 1–2). Baltimore: Paul H. Brookes Publishing Co.

Remington, B., Hastings, R.P., Kovshoff, H., degli Espinosa, F., Jahr, E., Brown, T., et al. (2007). Early intensive behavioral intervention: Outcomes for children with autism and their parents after two years. *American Journal on Mental Retardation, 112*(6), 418–438.

Rimland, B. (1964). *Infantile autism: The syndrome and its implications for a neural theory of behavior.* Appleton-Century-Crofts.

Schopler, E., Short, A., & Mesibov, G. (1989). Relation of behavioral treatment to "normal functioning": comment on Lovaas. *Journal of Consulting and Clinical Psychology, 57*(1), 162–164.

Skinner, B.F. (1938). Behavior of organisms. NY: Appleton Century Crofts, Inc.

Skinner, B.F. (1953). Science and human behavior. NY: Macmillan, Inc.

Smith, T., Groen, A., & Wynn, J. (2000). Randomized trial of intensive early intervention for children with pervasive developmental disorder. *American Journal on Mental Retardation, 105,* 269–285.

Sundberg, M. (2008). *Verbal Behavior Milestones Assessment and Placement Program.* Concord, CAA: Advancement of Verbal Behavior Press, Inc.

Sundberg, M.L. (2007). Verbal behavior. In J. O. Cooper, T. E. Heron, & W. L. Heward, *Applied behavior analysis* (2nd ed.) (pp. 526-547). Upper Saddle River, NJ: Merrill/Prentice Hall.

Thompson, T., & Hollon, S.D. (2008). *Behavioral and cognitive-behavioral interventions.* In M.H. Ebert, B. Nurcombe, P.T. Loosen, & J. Leckman (Eds.), *Current diagnosis and treatment: Psychiatry* (pp. 139-149). New York: McGraw Hill Medical.

Vygotsky, L. (1978). *Mind in society: The development of higher psychological processes.* Cambridge, MA: Harvard University Press.

Warren, S.F., Fey, M.E., & Yoder, P.J. (2007). Differential treatment intensity research: A missing link to creating optimally effective communication interventions. *Mental Retardation and Developmental Disabilities Research Reviews, 13*(1), 70–77.

Watson, J.B. (1913). Psychology as a behaviorist views it. *Psychological Review, 20,* 158–177.

7 Discrete Trial Intervention for Children with Limited Social and Language Skills and Intellectual Delays

with Beth Burggraff and Clover A. Anderson

"Practice is the best of all instructors."
—Publilius Syrus, *Maxim 439* (1894)

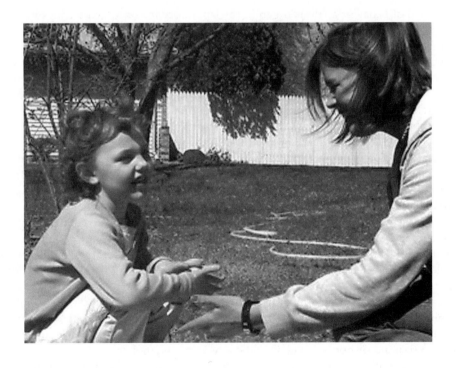

● ● ● ● ● ● ● ● ● ●

INTRODUCTION: PATRICK

Patrick, age 3½, had rosy cheeks and deep brown eyes that twinkled as he looked up at Clover, his senior behavior therapist. He was watching her attentively. Patrick had been diagnosed with Autistic Disorder and had little functional speech and poor joint attention, and he tended to play with toys repetitively, not imaginatively. He did not play with other children his age. He often engaged in *edging*, a form of visual self-stimulation, when he was not occupied by an adult. Patrick often had tantrums if his preferred activities were interrupted. Patrick had come to enjoy working with Clover and the other therapists. As he held a plastic saucer in his right hand, he painstakingly studied the cups on the right and a stack of saucers on the left that Clover had placed on the table before him. Clover said, "Patrick, put it with the same," as she handed him the toy saucer. He scanned from the cups to the saucers and back, and after hesitating briefly, he placed the saucer on the correct stack along with the other saucers. Clover said, "Great job, Patrick, you put it with the same!" and offered him a slice of apple, his favorite fruit snack.

● ● ● ● ● ● ● ● ● ●

Patrick is typical of children who often participate in Discrete Trial EIBI, also known as Discrete Trial Intervention (DTI). The strategy maximizes Patrick's success and the quick pace of the activity keeps him focused, preventing him from drifting off into self-stimulatory activities. In this chapter, we will discuss the theoretical foundation, setting, materials, procedures, and outcome measures involved in DTI.

DISCRETE TRIAL INTERVENTION PRINCIPLES AND ASSUMPTIONS

The field of behavior analysis began in the laboratory in controlled settings in which the experimenter arranged for a rewarding consequence, if and only if the subject made the correct response. In this setting, the subject's behavior became highly predictable. It was possible to induce the subject's responses to occur rapidly or slowly by turning on lights or playing tones that signaled different reinforcement conditions. The effects were precise and have been repeated in different laboratories throughout the world by different researchers many thousands of times. The learning principles involved were very robust and generalized.

In the 1960s, when Ivar Lovaas at UCLA began studying children with autism in clinical situations that were much less controlled than laboratory operant learning, he nonetheless looked to B.F. Skinner's laboratory model for ideas (Lovaas, 1967). He reasoned that, if it were possible to teach laboratory subjects to perform complex tasks, it should be possible to teach children with autism to perform important tasks, such as responding when spoken to, following directions, and perhaps even talking, using similar strategies. Lovaas was keenly aware that children are incredibly more complex and qualitatively different from the subjects studied in Skinner's laboratory, but he and his colleagues reasoned that *the same principles* should apply to children's learning but in more complex forms (Lovaas, Koegel, Simmons, & Long, 1973).

Laboratory learning almost never occurred in discrete trials in which a light or tone was presented, a single response occurred, and a reward (e.g., food) was provided. In the laboratory, the animal's behavior was called *free operant* because the subject was free to respond or not respond as it chose as it meandered around the experimental space, more like in the real world. (See Ferster, 1953, for further discussion.)

Nonetheless, the subject's behavior became increasingly affected by the consequences of its actions and the signal conditions indicating when and how its activities would be reinforced. Lovaas decided that it made sense to teach children with autism using the same operant principles, but in a series of discrete trials, i.e., stimulus-response-consequence, rather than in the free operant format, which is more like incidental teaching. A therapist who was seated across the table from the child, rather than lights or automated equipment, provided stimulus conditions and consequences. The stimuli were the therapists' or parents' voices, pictures and symbols on cards, three-dimensional objects, or—later in therapy—voices and actions of siblings and friends. Consequences included praise, hugs, preferred activities, and edible treats. As we shall see in succeeding sections, there were good reasons for Lovaas's decision to use a discrete trial format. But that choice also created challenges because not all children with autism had such severe disabilities as the first 7- to 9-year-olds with whom Lovaas initially worked at UCLA. In fact, most children with autism do not have severe disabilities. Let us first discuss Lovaas's DTI method, and later we will explore naturalistic interventions.

Stimulus-Response-Consequence

DTI is often an appropriate initial early intervention approach for children with ASDs who display little or no spoken language, display little social interest, have limited appropriate toy play, and display extensive nonfunctional ritualistic behavior (Maurice, 1996). Children like Patrick are usually not internally motivated by mastery of learning materials, such as being able to put together puzzles or stack toys, and often are unable to play with toys as they are intended. Learning occurs when a child makes a response in a given situation, such as Patrick putting the toy saucer with the other saucers but not the cups. That matching response is followed by a positive consequence, such as playing a tickle game, or in Patrick's case, enjoying a slice of apple. Children learn to do things that pay off for them. The DTI approach capitalizes on this tendency. A child is presented with relevant learning cues (e.g., a picture of Mom alongside a picture of Dad, and a teacher says, "Point to Mom") and the child responds selectively by pointing to the face with its unique "Mom" features but not the other familiar face with "Dad" features; then a reward is presented (e.g., tickles and praise such as "You're so smart, Helen!"). The reinforcer may be directly related to the task and situation, such as a sip of juice from the cup that the child had just selected, but in DTI that is not a requirement. A child is more likely to learn when he or she is highly motivated. In the case of Patrick, the therapist had already determined that Patrick greatly enjoyed chase games and physical play. The therapist made certain she had not provided physical "horseplay" with Patrick for the past hour or so before beginning therapy. As a result, the opportunity to play a tickle game with his caregiver was especially motivating. Patrick was "raring to go."

Learning Is Incremental

A second assumption is that learning new skills is incremental and requires many repetitions. Initial skill acquisition may be painstakingly slow at times—indeed, so slow that it may appear little progress is being made. Children with autism, especially younger kids with more limited skills, usually do not display "aha!" learning experiences in which they suddenly appear to "get it." Instead, "steady as she goes" is the DTI motto. Children with very limited skills must repeat this stimulus-response-consequence sequence frequently, on a given learning occasion (e.g., Tuesday morning at 10 a.m.) as well as across learning opportunities (e.g., over successive days and weeks). This ensures that gains that have been made are consolidated and aren't lost through disuse or interfering experience. By inspecting graphs of learning of new skills over weeks and months (Figure 7.1), parents and teachers can see that, though there may be occasional plateaus and reversals, their child is actually making solid progress overall, albeit in baby steps that are often not obvious from one day to the next. In the case of the graph in Figure 7.1, the goal was for the child to establish eye contact with the listener when addressing him or her to recruit his or her attention.

Create Learning Opportunities—Don't Wait for the Child to Initiate

If one were to wait until a child like Patrick showed interest in looking at pictures of people's faces, in most instances it would be necessary to wait a very long time. Some children may never spontaneously show interest in looking at faces or in other important learning activities. Within a DTI intervention format, the therapist or teacher structures learning opportunities that maintain the child's interest and keeps her or him actively engaged on topic. This is accomplished by presenting learning opportunities in a series of reasonably paced discrete trials: in other words, stimulus-response-reinforcer sequences, usually in the same setting, using the same learning materials (at least initially), and following the same spoken and gestural instructions. A trial typically lasts several seconds but not much longer. Although many neurotypical children may become bored if the same learning materials are presented repeatedly, children with autism often thrive on repetition of familiar stimuli and procedures. The DTI procedure capitalizes on the fact that children with autism prefer predictable routines. Interpolated between groups of learning trials are free play opportunities employing materials in which the child has previously shown interest, such as cause-and-effect toys (e.g., jack-in-the-box) or crawling through an expandable nylon tunnel.

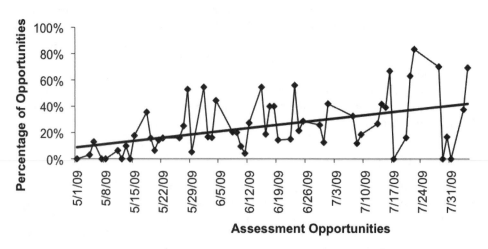

Figure 7.1. Diagram showing slow, steady progress during Discrete Trial Intervention (DTI). Over the course of several weeks, the child was learning how to recruit adult attention by establishing eye contact when speaking to adults.

Overcoming Self-Stimulation and Compulsive Routines

Many children with ASDs devote an inordinate amount of time to repetitive, nonfunctional self-stimulatory activities, such as edging, finger flicking, or picking up toys and repetitively dropping them on the floor, which is a persistent early developmental behavioral pattern. It may be difficult to interrupt these highly fixed routines, which, if intruded upon, can be followed by a meltdown. *Edging* refers to visually scanning along the straight edges of objects or features of a room, such as ceiling molding, lines in the carpeting, or window frames. *Finger flicking* is a repetitive movement of fingers before the child's eyes, often while moving his or her head from side to side in a rhythmic fashion. A father once told me he wasn't concerned about his child's self-stimulation behaviors and that he thinks his son will outgrow them. But such self-stimulatory behavior can significantly interfere with a child's focusing on the relevant learning materials and tends to expand to fill an increasing proportion of the child's unoccupied time. At times, some self-stimulatory responses, such as pulling at one's own hair or repeatedly slapping hands together, can gradually mutate into self-injury, such as face slapping or banging hands against hard surfaces. Self-stimulation can be reduced by providing clear instructions and using highly valued reinforcers with high frequency for participation and correct responding. The more actively engaged the child becomes, the less frequent and intense self-stimulatory behavior and the greater skill improvements. Functional activities eventually replace most self-stimulatory behavior.

Coping with Attention Problems

Most children with autism have significant attention problems. Some may be diagnosed with ADHD was well as autism. At intervention outset, some young children on the autism spectrum may look at a stimulus presented to them by their teacher, parent, or therapist only for a few seconds. When we began working with her, 4-year-old Jesi, who was diagnosed with Autistic Disorder, sat in her chair and glanced at a picture of candy and another picture of a piece of fruit for no more than 1 to 3 seconds—insufficient time to be certain of what she was seeing. However, once she discovered she could have the item the therapist named if she touched the corresponding picture with her finger, she began paying greater attention and looked more carefully for longer intervals at the choice stimuli. If the teacher or therapist makes it worthwhile for the child to look more closely and pay attention, most children with autism can learn to do so, and for longer intervals.

Addressing Stimulus Overselectivity

Children with autism tend to focus on a single aspect of a visual stimulus (e.g., focus on the mouth or the hairline on a picture of a face and pay no attention to the rest of the face, including the person's eyes). This tendency lends itself to the child's focusing on unimportant aspects of learning materials. This phenomenon, called *stimulus overselectivity,* creates challenges for teaching visual discrimination skills. Specific DTI intervention techniques are employed to ensure that the child is attending to relevant aspects of learning stimuli, not only to those that initially capture their interest (Dickson, Wang, Lombard, & Dube, 2006; Schreibman, Koegel, & Craig, 1977). The usual teaching procedure involves having the child select the correct picture that matches the sample (e.g., Mom vs. Dad). One technique for reducing overselectivity requires the child to touch the sample (e.g., the picture of Mom) or name the picture (e.g., says "Mom") before choosing the correct matching picture (Mom vs. Dad). The DTI procedure facilitates the child's learning to more systematically look at learning materials before choosing the matching stimulus.

Provide Frequent Reinforcement for Participation and Correct Responding

Having responded once to an adult request, such as "Point to Mom," when presented with photos of both Mom and Dad, the child may attempt to immediately leave the therapy or teaching situation. The child may rise from the table and run across the room and resist being guided back to the therapy table. That makes it difficult to provide sufficient practice with a given skill so that the child has an opportunity to learn appropriate responses to important social, cognitive, or communicative stimuli. The parent or therapist may find her- or himself chasing the resistant child and attempting to return to the intervention situation. But being chased by an adult can inadvertently become a reinforcing activity that interferes with learning. One must work diligently at providing very frequent reinforcement for the child's remaining engaged. By providing powerful reinforcers and interpolating short, child-selected play activities with positively reinforced learning opportunities, it is often possible to keep very distractible children, who tend to elope from the learning situation, engaged for progressively longer time intervals. If chase games are reinforcing for a given child, it is better that they are used as reinforcers for participating in learning activities. Once a child has performed a specified number of receptive matching responses (e.g., pointing to pictures or objects), the therapist then plays a chase game with the child.

Fear of, and Resistance to, New Materials or Procedures

Perhaps the most difficult aspect of providing learning opportunities for some young children with autism, especially lower functioning youngsters with Autistic Disorder, is their tendency to assiduously avoid new learning activities or materials. Nadia, age 3, screamed, pulled away, and hit her therapist whenever a new toy, game, or book was included in therapy, even one that seemed quite similar to those with which she was accustomed. Children with ASDs often shove away learning materials, escape from the situation, and throw themselves on the floor, flailing. Some hit, kick, or bite caregivers or strike or scratch themselves in the face when presented with a new learning activity, no matter how benign. Many reinforced desensitization trials over numerous sessions may be required to overcome the child's phobic response to new stimuli and promote the inclusion of new learning materials. Repeating trials and rewarding the child for tolerating new materials very gradually introduced will generally lead to acceptance. Early in therapy, Nadia required from 2 to 4 weeks to tolerate each new toy or book introduced into therapy.

Problems with Following the Child's Lead or Assuming Learning Is Inherently Rewarding

The combination of challenging characteristics of some children with severe autism and lesser cognitive ability, and the nature of the underlying learning processes, create difficulties for early intervention approaches that assume the therapist or teacher can make significant learning gains by following the child's lead, or that a child with an ASD will be inherently excited about the opportunity to learn. Many children with

Autistic Disorder and some with PDD-NOS do best if therapy begins in a more structured format and employs repetitive procedures and materials that are inherent in a DTI approach. For the remainder of the chapter we discuss the learning principles, setting, materials, and procedures employed in the DTI approach. The chapter concludes with sample intervention plans and child outcomes.

ROOTS IN APPLIED BEHAVIOR ANALYSIS PRINCIPLES

The intervention practices employed in DTI grow out of extensive behavior analysis laboratory research on learning as well as ABA research in clinical and educational settings, which is beyond the scope of this discussion. In order for readers to use the principles and techniques in the following section in working with a child with autism, they must have considerable supervised experience with youngsters with autism and have completed a college-level course that includes principles of ABA and equivalent in pre- and in-service training.

Principles of ABA guide the details of specific interventions (e.g., differential reinforcement, discrimination learning, type and scheduling or reinforcement, shaping and chaining, stimulus fading) in the day-to-day practice of DTI (Cooper, Heron, & Heward, 2007). These basic science behavioral principles used in autism intervention, as well as in many other educational and clinical applications, are comparable to physiology principles that underlie diagnosis and treatment in various areas of medicine. ABA is not the same thing as DTI; DTI is one of many *practical* applications of ABA principles and techniques.

Data Intensity

DTI is very data intensive, often with trial-by-trial records of whether the child's response was correct (e.g., child claps hands) following a given stimulus (e.g., "Do this while clapping hands"), the degree of prompting required (e.g., an assistant gently guides the child's hands into a clapping motion or only gestures with a point), and suggested adjustments in the procedure on the next session (e.g., gradually reduce prompts) based on child outcome measures. Data are graphed regularly and reviewed by all team members, including the child's parents, at weekly or biweekly meetings. Intervention decisions are made in large part based on data indicating a procedure is producing learning, or is not, in which case the procedure is changed. A typical DTI intervention plan for a 2- to 4-year-old child with Autistic Disorder may include 8–10 goals, which are often broken down into smaller subobjectives. Progress on each is monitored regularly.

Setting

The physical setting within which DTI intervention takes place may vary, but the most common occurs with the child and therapist seated across from one another at a child-sized table, often in a spare bedroom, a seldom-used family room, or a study. The setting should be as uncluttered as possible, quiet, and devoid of distractions such as television, music devices, video games, and so forth. Most highly appealing play materials are stored on shelves or in covered storage bins or behind closed doors or curtains to avoid competition for the child's attention. Parents are asked to turn off or turn down televisions, music players, computer audio output, or other sources of distracting sounds emanating from nearby rooms such as a sibling's bedroom. Mobiles, wall hangings, or other decorative items are discouraged if they include shiny, moving components, such as beads, reflective materials, or sequins, which are often very distracting to children with ASDs.

A family with whom we recently worked had a large flat-screen television monitor in the recreation room that served as the therapy room. Though the television was turned off during therapy, the black screen was highly reflective and very distracting to the 3-year-old child with autism, who moved his head from side to side as he stared at his reflection in the television screen. We covered the screen with a quilt from a nearby sofa to reduce this distraction. Windows facing outdoors are often covered with blinds or translucent curtains if they provide a view of distracting outdoor activities nearby, such as a trampoline or swimming pool with siblings or neighborhood children playing.

It is appropriate to place colorful learning-related posters on therapy room walls, such as letters of the alphabet, images of animals, seasons of the year, or nature scenes. Posters related to a child's obsessions or fixed interests should be avoided, as these can encourage their ritualistic behavior. Linda, a bright child with Asperger syndrome, is fixated on dogs, insisting on talking with everyone she meets about dogs and asking questions about their dog's name, breed, color, size, age, and so forth, often well beyond a point that it is appropriate. Photos or images of dogs were excluded from the primary learning areas in which Linda's intervention most often occurred, though she encountered dogs when on community therapy outings. Initially, siblings and pets can be excluded from the therapy area to minimize distractions. Once the child with ASD has become accustomed to the learning routines, family members, friends, and pets are incorporated into therapy.

Materials

Supplies and learning materials are typically kept in a locked cabinet in the therapy room, and perishable edibles may be stored in a nearby refrigerator (e.g., for fresh fruit or beverages) out of the child's reach. Among the most important supplies is the child's *program book,* which contains written copies of each intervention procedure addressing each objective—including the materials needed, the procedures to be followed, and the data to be recorded. Within the program book on the first page is a copy of the child's descriptive information: name, date of birth, date of last diagnostic assessment, name and address of the professional who conducted the assessment, parents' names and addresses, telephone numbers, e-mail addresses, child's diagnosis, primary physician, medications and dosages the child is receiving, school contacts, and the name of another adult to contact in case of an emergency (Figure 7.2).

At the top of the program book's first page—in bold letters in a large font, all capitals—is an indication of any allergies for which the child has been diagnosed by a physician, such as peanuts, eggs, milk, soy, wheat, or gluten; and emergency instructions in case of an allergy attack. Below the allergy warning, on a separate line, is a list of any other significant medical conditions the child has, such as epilepsy, diabetes, or asthma, and monitoring instructions and medications or other treatments for those conditions, so that the staff is aware of possible medical problems or emergencies. Behavior therapy or instructional staff are typically not involved in conducting medical monitoring (e.g., blood sugar measurement) or administering treatments, but should be aware of signs of a health problem, such as difficulty breathing, signs of high blood sugar, or the onset of a seizure, so that they can immediately alert the child's parents or other primary caregiver.

Contact Information Sheet

Client: Billy Smith   **Date of birth:** 9/14/06

Parents: William and Joan Smith,
            10829 Whitfield Lane, Middletown, MN
            (555-344-0799)

PEANUT ALLERGY

- Billy Smith is allergic to peanuts or products containing peanuts or peanut oil. If he begins showing allergic symptoms (e.g., hives, flushing, choking) after consuming any food or beverage, his parents should be immediately notified and he should receive an EpiPen injection. **If Billy has difficulty breathing, call 911.**

- Billy receives Depakote for epilepsy (see below).

Diagnosis: Autistic Disorder 299.9

Primary care physician: Marilyn Johnson, M.D.; Suburban Clinic, Middletown, MN (555-232-1900)

Medications: EpiPen Jr 0.15mg epinephrine injection; Depakote 15mg/day; Miralax 3oz 2/day; Multivitamin 1 wafer per day

Special diet: No peanuts, peanut products, or items containing peanut oil

School: Middletown Early Childhood Special Education Program; Linda Olson, M.A., special education teacher (555-652-1000)

Social worker: Marie Atwood, Clayton County Social Services (555-651-1000)

Additional emergency adult contact: Evelyn Smith (Billy's paternal aunt) (555-692-0856)

Figure 7.2.   Sample child health, family, and agency contact information form for a program book.

In subsequent pages, the program book contains contacts for all therapy staff and the individualized treatment plan or individualized education program (IEP) and forms on which progress is recorded, beginning with the goal at the top of each page, the materials required, and a brief summary of the intervention procedure (Figure 7.3).

A separate section, indicated by a tab in the program book, contains forms on which narrative *progress notes* are recorded chronologically, including objectives on which the child worked, progress made, problems encountered, and suggestions for the next therapist or teacher who continues intervention on that objective.

During an initial home visit, parents are provided with a list of potential reinforcers on which to indicate what their son or daughter enjoys, divided into categories: 1) activities, 2) social, 3) tangible, and 4) consumable (Figure 7.4). For each item on the list, parents are asked to indicate whether the item is preferred, of intermediate preference, disliked, or is of unknown interest to the child. Any items the parents wish to exclude are crossed out on the list. After a discussion with the parents, typically therapy begins with two to three reinforcer items from each of these four categories to provide some variability. Parents are encouraged to purchase only items that are consumable or most highly preferred until it is determined which are most effective. Tangibles (e.g., preferred toys) and materials used in specific activities (e.g., a mini-trampoline) can often be borrowed from relatives or friends or purchased at a thrift store. As much as possible, parents are asked not to make those

Individual Treatment Plan

Child's name: Zachary Jones   Date of birth: 10-26-02

Date of plan: December 15, 2008

Goal heading: Follow picture schedule

ITP goal area: Restricted or stereotyped behaviors

Baseline probe date: December 15, 2008

Objective introduced: December 15, 2008   **Objective mastered:** May 2009

Behavioral objective:
Zachary will follow a picture schedule with 1 prompt or less, for up to 5 pictures, without protest, 80% of opportunities across 3 consecutive probe assessments.

Treatment procedure(s):

1. Prepare picture schedule of 5 activities (begin with 2 of the 5).
2. Show Zachary or have him place picture on schedule.
3. Record as a *correct* if Zachary follows schedule with one prompt or less without protest.
4. If he protests or needs to be redirected or reminded of the schedule more than one time, document as an *incorrect*.
5. If Zachary follows schedule independently without protest, reinforce with praise, a treat, and access to preferred game at conclusion of schedule!
6. We will systematically add pictures on the schedule, starting with two pictures.

Work on this skill with a variety of activities. If we need more schedule pictures, please record on the treatment update page.

Additional information:

Prompting: Start with most-to-least prompting hierarchy (e.g., physical, partial physical, movement, modeling) and continue to follow through with schedule.

Incorrect response: Elopement, verbal protests, engaging in challenging behaviors

Figure 7.3.   Individual treatment plan goal for a child receiving Discrete Trial Intervention (DTI). The purpose is to reduce tangential, nonfunctional repetitive behavior by providing a picture schedule to reduce ambiguity and maintain on-task activities.

items available to the child at other times between therapy sessions so they retain their special value to the child during therapy.

Stimulus materials used during therapy sessions are individualized and planned during an initial individualized treatment plan or IEP meeting.

Procedures

Home-based therapy services usually last about 2 hours per day, 5 days per week, and time gradually increases over a month to 6 weeks, to approximately 30 hours per week (e.g.,

Reinforcer Inventory

Child's name: _____   Date of birth: _____

Parent name(s): _____   Date of plan: _____

Therapist name(s): _____

Instructions to parents: For each item listed, indicate how much you think your child enjoys or likely enjoys the activity or item listed with a check mark. *Not at all; Some; Quite a bit; Very much.* If you don't want your child to have access to any item, cross it out.

Instructions to therapists: Select the two highest ranking items in B, C, and D, and three highest ranking items in A and E to use initially as reinforcers. Change reinforcers frequently to avoid rigid routines. To maintain some novelty, rotate out one item in each category each week and substitute the next-highest ranking item in each category.

	Not at all	Some	Quite a bit	Very much
A. Social				
Being given horseback rides	___	___	___	___
Being read to	___	___	___	___
Being tickled	___	___	___	___
Playing chase games	___	___	___	___
Helping Dad	___	___	___	___
Helping Mom	___	___	___	___
Playing "I See..."	___	___	___	___
Playing "Simon Says"	___	___	___	___
Playing "Red Light/Green Light"	___	___	___	___
Playing with brother or sister	___	___	___	___
Singing songs with hand motions (e.g., "Itsy Bitsy Spider")	___	___	___	___
Taking care of pet	___	___	___	___
Other _____	___	___	___	___
B. Fine Motor Activities and Crafts				
Soap for blowing bubbles	___	___	___	___
Cars and trucks	___	___	___	___
Car ramps	___	___	___	___
Computer time (e.g., video games)	___	___	___	___
Container filled with beans or rice	___	___	___	___
Crayons and coloring books	___	___	___	___
Doctor kit	___	___	___	___
Dollhouse	___	___	___	___
Dress-up clothing	___	___	___	___
Farmhouse kit	___	___	___	___
Felt-tip markers	___	___	___	___
Felt, fabric, safety scissors, and glue	___	___	___	___

(continued)

Figure 7.4. Reinforcer Inventory for program book.

	Not at all	Some	Quite a bit	Very much
Legos	_____	_____	_____	_____
Light-up spinners	_____	_____	_____	_____
Play-Doh	_____	_____	_____	_____
Preferred video	_____	_____	_____	_____
Puzzles (peg, inset, interlocking)	_____	_____	_____	_____
Slime	_____	_____	_____	_____
Squishy toys/balls	_____	_____	_____	_____
Rubber stamps/Scrapbooking	_____	_____	_____	_____
Trains	_____	_____	_____	_____
Water color/tempera paint	_____	_____	_____	_____
Water table	_____	_____	_____	_____
Other _____	_____	_____	_____	_____

C. Tangibles

	Not at all	Some	Quite a bit	Very much
Privilege coupons	_____	_____	_____	_____
Special toys/trinkets	_____	_____	_____	_____
Stamps	_____	_____	_____	_____
Stars	_____	_____	_____	_____
Stickers	_____	_____	_____	_____
Toiletries (preferred soap, shampoo)	_____	_____	_____	_____
Tokens and token boards	_____	_____	_____	_____
Trading cards	_____	_____	_____	_____
Other _____	_____	_____	_____	_____

D. Gross Motor Activities

	Not at all	Some	Quite a bit	Very much
Ball pit	_____	_____	_____	_____
Bean bag (or ring) toss	_____	_____	_____	_____
Gross motor games (tag, ball)	_____	_____	_____	_____
Mini-trampoline	_____	_____	_____	_____
Treadmill	_____	_____	_____	_____
Tricycle (or bicycle for older children)	_____	_____	_____	_____
Swimming	_____	_____	_____	_____
Swinging	_____	_____	_____	_____
Other _____	_____	_____	_____	_____

E. Edibles and Beverages

	Not at all	Some	Quite a bit	Very much
Animal crackers	_____	_____	_____	_____
Ants on a Log (low-fat, low-salt peanut butter spread in celery sticks with raisins sprinkled on top, cut into 1-inch lengths)	_____	_____	_____	_____
Baked low-salt potato, tortilla, or other chips	_____	_____	_____	_____

Reinforcer Inventory *(continued)*

	Not at all	Some	Quite a bit	Very much
Dried fruit (raisins, apples, pears, apricots); cut larger fruit into smaller pieces	___	___	___	___
Edamame (soybeans in pods); boil in chicken or beef broth to add flavor and cool	___	___	___	___
Fresh pieces of fruit (grapes, apples, pears)	___	___	___	___
Frozen grapes, strawberries, or banana chunks	___	___	___	___
Fruit roll-ups cut into pieces	___	___	___	___
Light salted popcorn without butter	___	___	___	___
Low-salt pretzels (small sticks or swirls)	___	___	___	___
Mini-rice cakes	___	___	___	___
Pure sugarless fruit juice and carbonated water or mineral water (50:50)	___	___	___	___
String cheese cut into pieces	___	___	___	___
Other _____	___	___	___	___

increasing from 10 to 15 to 20 to 25 to 30 hours per week). A typical intervention program would call for stabilizing on a schedule—for example, intervention may occur on Monday, Wednesday, and Friday from 8:30 a.m. to 11:30 a.m. and 2 p.m. to 4 p.m.; and Tuesday and Thursday, 9:30 a.m. to noon and 2:30 p.m. to 5 p.m. (Figure 7.5). This allows time for lunch, potty breaks, and a nap. Each therapist would work with such a child approximately 8–9 hours per week in 2- or 3-hour shifts. This strategy has several advantages:

· It is not helpful if a child will only exhibit a particular skill for their favorite therapist, teaching staff member, or one parent but not the other. The child needs to become accustomed to engaging in appropriate behavior in the presence of several adults to encourage generalization.

· The child will be less likely to lose interest if the adult working with him or her differs within each day (e.g., Beth may work with the child from 8:30 a.m. to 11:30 a.m. and Aaron may provide therapy from 2 p.m. to 4 p.m.).

· Conducting individual behavior therapy with a young child with autism over an extended time period is extremely demanding for therapy staff members, especially if the child exhibits significant challenging behavior. The therapist must constantly be at the top of his or her game in order to maintain upbeat demeanor and not eventually burn out. By limiting therapists to 2- to 3-hour shifts and changing children with whom they work between mornings and afternoons, staff members are able to retain their freshness and enthusiasm with each child.

Weekly Schedule

Child's name: __Jesi__   Week of: __March 14__

Day/date	Monday	# HRS	Tuesday	# HRS	Wednesday	# HRS	Thursday	# HRS	Friday	HRS
8:00 AM										
9:00 AM	Sue		Anika		Sue		Meredith		Anika	
	9am–12pm		9am–12pm		9am–12pm		9am–12pm		9am–12pm	
10:00 AM										
11:00 AM										
		3.00		3.00		3.00		3.00		3.00
12:00 PM	Meredith				Meredith					
	12:30–3:00pm				12:30–3:00pm					
1:00 PM			Vicki				Anika		Sue	
			1–4pm				1–3pm		1–4pm	
2:00 PM										
		2.50					2.50		2.00	
3:00 PM						3.00				3.00
	Beth						Vicki			
4:00 PM	3:30–5:30pm						3:30–5:30pm			
	Family skills									
5:00 PM		2.00						2.00		

Figure 7.5. Jesi's typical weekly schedule once therapy services had been ramped up and stabilized. Therapy is typically scheduled between 8 a.m. and 5:30 p.m. on Monday through Friday. (Some parents and their staff negotiate weekend sessions as well, but that is not typical. Key: HRS = hours)

The First Few Weeks

The first 2 to 3 weeks of the ramp-up process is usually devoted to familiarizing the child with each therapist with whom he or she will be working and desensitizing the child to having new adults in their home. This process, also sometimes called *rapport building, pairing,* or *the child's game,* associates each therapist with positive experiences (e.g., playing with the child while providing access to desired reinforcers but without making demands on the child). This reduces the child's resistance and engenders trust that this adult will not ask him or her to do anything that is too difficult or too disturbing. Therapy staff members use this period to develop an inventory of things the child chooses to do spontaneously and things the child avoids or appears to dislike. As the child spontaneously plays with a ball or toy cars, the therapist may say something like, "Liz rolls the ball," or "Brian drives the car," simply describing what the child is doing. The child becomes familiar with each therapist's voice and with his or her appearance, gestures, and movements. The child's initial apprehensiveness is largely eliminated. By the end of about 2 to 3 weeks, when therapists arrive at the family's home, most children with an ASD run up to them as they enter the front door and take their hand, or hold up their arms to be picked up and held. The child comes to think of each therapist as a nice adult who comes to his or her house to play. When this begins to happen, the next stage of intervention begins.

Assessment

Unlike most typical psychological or educational assessments, EIBI uses criterion-referenced assessments rather than norm-referenced assessments (Bond, 1996). *Norm-referenced tests,* such as the Wechsler Preschool and Primary Scale of Intelligence (WPPSI; Wechsler, 2002) or the Vineland Adaptive Behavior Scales–II (VABS-II; Sparrow, Cicchetti, & Balla, 2005), give a child's scores in various domains in relation to other children their age, either stated as an age equivalent (e.g., 18 months) or a percentile rank (e.g., 27th percentile). The latter rank indicates that 73% of the child's peers score higher on that scale. These tests do not prescribe specific cognitive, adaptive, language, or social skills that should be taught or the focus of therapy. *Criterion-referenced tests* measure a large number of individual skills (e.g., imitates simple hand movements) that, taken together, comprise most of the skills that a child should exhibit to function similarly to their peers in a given age range. The Assessment of Basic Language and Learning Skills–Revised (ABLLS-R; Partington, 2007) and the Verbal Behavior Milestones Assessment and Placement Program (VB-MAPP; Sundberg, 2008) are criterion-referenced assessments for children with autism. Each skill within a given scale, such as simple motor imitation, is scored as being demonstrated, and with what degree of prompting and consistency. This type of information does not permit comparison with same-age peers; in other words, it does not provide a percentile rank. But it *does* indicate which specific skills within each domain a child currently demonstrates and which he or she lacks. For example, the VB-MAPP includes 900 skills covering the 16 domains. The milestones are broken into three developmental levels: 0–18 months, 18–30 months, and 30–48 months. The scores for each skill are approximately balanced across each level. There are five items and five possible points for each skill area. Once these "milestones" have been assessed and the general skill level has been established, the task analysis, which is part of the assessment, can provide further information about a particular child to inform intervention planning (Sundberg, 2008). Mark Sundberg, the VB-MAPP's developer, points out that it is also important to know why a child is unable to perform a given skill. The VB-MAPP Barriers Assessment is designed to identify 22 different learning and language acquisition barriers. Scores in these domains and knowledge of possible barriers, together with other parent and therapist concerns, provide the foundation for developing an initial treatment plan, including priorities.

On Figure 7.6, Jesi's baseline ABLLS scores (shown in dark squares) for the first nine scales most relevant to home-based intervention indicated she had very limited skills in cooperation, visual performance, and requests. On most of the remaining scales, Jesi was unable to perform at the basal levels.

A VB-MAPP for a child with similar skills, Robin, provided by Dr. Mark Sundberg, reveals somewhat more strengths in receptive language, visual perceptual matching, play, and imitation in Level 1 skills (0–18 months), but similar lack of skills above the 18-month range (Figure 7.7).

Beginning Therapy

Jesi scored 1.15 on the Autism Intervention Responsiveness Scale (AIRS™; see Chapter 4, Figure 4.1). Children scoring below 1.4 generally profit most from a DTI approach. One of the first requests made of Jesi was to come to the table and sit in her chair. This is usually stated by the adult: "Jesi, come sit," accompanied by pointing to the seat of the chair and a movement of the adult's hand downward with the palm facing down. Many children with Autistic Disorder do not comply with this request. After two or three attempts distributed over several minutes, the therapist places one hand in the middle of the child's back or on his shoulder and with the other, points to the chair and says, "Jesi, come sit," as he or she gently guides the child to the chair. The moment the child is seated, the child is praised—"Good job, thanks for sitting!"—and an edible reward, such as sugarless candy or baked potato chips, is given to the child, depending on what the parents indicated would be most rewarding and which items the child seemed to enjoy during the initial rapport-building period. A small toy that previously has been of interest to the child during the "child's game" is resting on the table in front of the child, who is encouraged to push the car or something similar. After the child has been seated for a minute or two and has touched and/or played with the toy, he or she is invited to sit on the floor and play with familiar materials that were of interest during previous "pairing" sessions. Following 5 minutes or so of free play, the instruction "Come sit" will be repeated again, accompanied by pointing. If the child doesn't sit as requested, she or he is guided gently, repeating the reinforcement procedure as before. If the child runs away or is highly resistant, the therapist stops making the request, waits a few minutes, and then resumes making the request. During the 5-minute periods between successive "Come sit" practice sessions, the child will be encouraged to sit on the floor and roll a ball back and forth with the therapist, with ample praise for doing so. Very gradually, small requests are made of the child when he or she is seated at the table, largely based on what he or she already had done during pairing. It is preferable to begin by requesting the child to do something he or she already likes to do. If the child gets up and walks away, the therapist waits and then invites him or her to sit at the table again to play with a preferred toy.

On the first 2-hour session, typically a child beginning therapy has 20 to 30 "come sit" trials. Usually toward the end of the first or second session, the child is beginning to take his or her seat at least part of the time following the verbal and gestural prompt, without manual guidance. Once the child is sitting reliably most of the time when

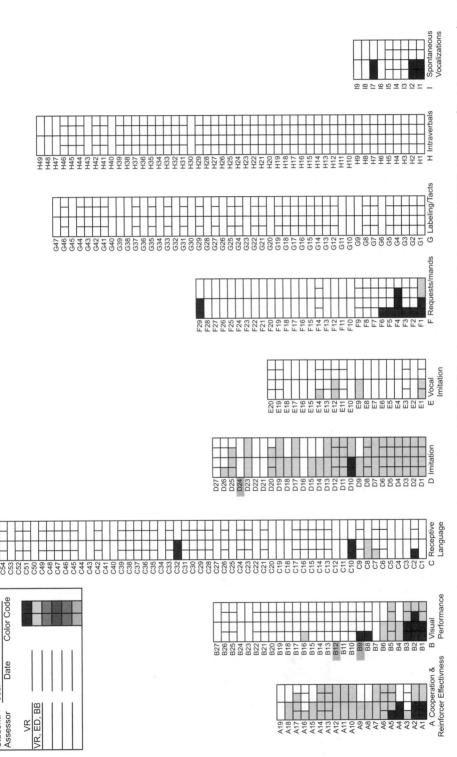

Figure 7.6. Jesi's baseline Assessment of Basic Language and Learning—Revised (ABLLS-R) Skill tracking system. (From Partington, J.W. [2007]. *Assessment of Basic Language and Learning Skills-Revised [ABLLS-R]*. Walnut Creek, CA: The Behavior Analysts, Inc.; adapted by permission.)

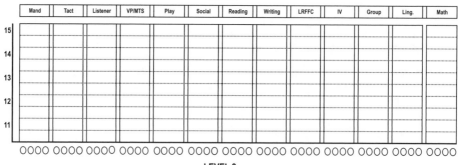

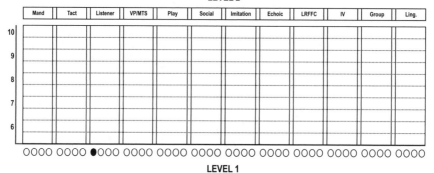

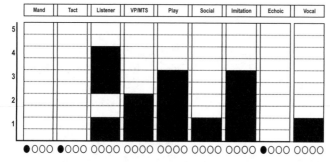

Figure 7.7.   Sample Verbal Behavior Milestones Assessment and Placement Program (VB-MAPP) baseline skills measure for a younger child with autism who has limited cognitive, language, and social skills. (From http://www.mark sundberg.com; reprinted by permission.)

requested, motor imitation learning typically begins. The therapist seated across from the child calls his or her name, waits for him or her to look, tells the child to "do this," and then claps his or her hands. An assistant or parent is standing behind the child and guides him or her hands together in a clapping motion. Initially, every time the child approximates the therapist's movement, a reinforcer (e.g., a small piece of fresh fruit) is immediately delivered, combined with praise (e.g., "Good clapping, Sarah"). If the child resists or cries, the person assisting releases the child's hands for several seconds, and then the instruction "Do this" is repeated, and the child's hands are guided together in a clapping motion. Resistance generally diminishes as the child discovers that nothing bad is going to happen and that he or she receives treats when seated at the table "playing" with the therapist.

Within and across sessions, the number of discrete trials is gradually increased as the child tolerates being seated and attending for progressively longer time intervals. Within any given session, if the child begins to be fussy, perhaps protesting, the number of repetitions is reduced and interpolated play periods lengthened. The goal is to keep the child positively engaged as long as possible without exceeding his or her tolerance. Always try to end the session on a positive note.

● ● ● ● ● ● ● ● ● ●

JESI: A CHILD WHO THRIVED ON DISCRETE TRIAL INTERVENTION

Jesi had just turned 4 years old when we first met her. Her striking persimmon–colored hair contrasted sharply with her hazel eyes, which shifted from light brown to a golden green, depending on her mood. She had freckles of varying sizes on her face, arms, and hands, reminiscent of Anne in *Anne of Green Gables* (Montgomery, 1908). She had been diagnosed with Autistic Disorder 18 months earlier. During my initial diagnostic observation, Jesi frenetically ricocheted around the room while making "eee-eee" sounds, stopping periodically to pick up a toy and then throwing it. She did not respond when spoken to, though at times she spontaneously oriented toward her mother. She did not imitate motor movements or speech or show interest in interacting with the adults in the room. She spoke a few inarticulate words, but they were not directed toward people. During a subsequent home observation, Jesi climbed on an end table, jumped, and bounced on the sofa. She resisted adult requests like "Jesi, come sit!" by running away, screaming and crying. Jesi's family had recently moved from Texas to Minnesota. On her bedroom wall was a plaque that read, "Dear Lord, please tell Mom that cowgirls don't take baths, they just dust off," which seemed especially apt for energetic Jesi. After conducting a detailed skills assessment and an inventory of Jesi's likes and dislikes, our therapy team initiated intensive home-based behavior therapy using a DTI approach. Her progress was initially slow, but with time her skill development accelerated. After 9 months of 30-hour-per-week therapy, I invited Terra, Jesi's mother, to share her thoughts about Jesi's and her family's experience with EIBI, which are presented later in this chapter.

Let's look again at Figure 7.5, which shows Jesi's typical weekly therapy schedule totaling 32 hours of planned time. Note that sessions never exceed 3 hours or fall short of 2 hours. This provides sufficient time for Jesi to warm up to therapy activities without exceeding her attention span and her tolerance for learning demands. Therapy involves three behavior therapists and one senior behavior therapist who work with Jesi's parents as well as with Jesi to help generalize new skills.

Individual Treatment Plan

Child: Jesi   **ITP Date**: 11/5/08

Objective heading: Increased motor imitation Skills

ITP goal area: Socialization

Baseline probe date: 11/10/08

Objective introduced: 11/10/08

Objective mastered: April 2009

Behavioral objective: When Jesi is asked to imitate an action modeled by an adult, both with objects and without, she will do so for 25 different actions, 80% of the time on three consecutive assessment opportunities with at least two caregivers.

Treatment procedure(s):

S^D 1: "Do this" (where Jesi and practitioner use identical sets of objects)
R: Jesi imitates the action exactly as the practitioner presented it to her.

Exemplars

Take Legos apart	Feed doll
Hold phone to ear	Brush hair
Put pizza on plate	Roll Play-Doh
Scribble with marker	Put coin in bank
Push car	Kiss doll
Put on hat	Open book
Put block in bucket	Drink from cup

S^D 2: "Do this" (where Jesi imitates an action presented by the practitioner without the use of objects)
R: Jesi imitates the action exactly as the practitioner presented it to her.

Exemplars

Clap	Sit down
Put your arms up	Give an item
Turn around	Put an item on/in
Jump	Open the door
Throw this away	Clean up
Blow a kiss	
Get a tissue	
Give me five	
Stomp your feet	
Wave	
Shut the door	
Turn on the light	
Color	

Figure 7.8. Sample Individual Treatment Plan for Jesi: Objective and suggested intervention procedures for increased motor imitation skills, one of Jesi's first socialization goals. (Key: S^D, Discriminative Stimulus; R, Response).

Jesi's Intervention Objectives

Figure 7.8 is an example of a socialization goal for Jesi from her individualized treatment plan. Jesi also had numerous other objectives as part of her intervention plan. A partial list is presented here:

1. Increases the number of Jesi's spontaneous PECS and verbal requests
2. Increased motor imitation
3. Requests a break
4. Follows a picture schedule
5. Increasingly imitates video modeling
6. Matches objects and pictures
7. Increasingly tolerates noises using headphones
8. Verbally imitates
9. Increasingly tolerates time delay
10. Increasingly tolerates denial

Jesi's Sample Outcomes

Jesi's skills were typically learned very slowly in the beginning, and then after 3 or 4 months they began improving more rapidly. Figure 7.9a and b presents graphs showing Jesi's progress with motor imitation and matching objects to pictures.

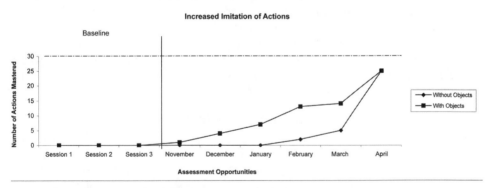

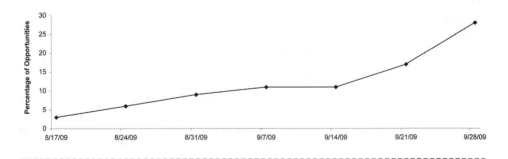

Figure 7.9. Graphic records of Jesi's progress in a) learning imitation of actions, and b) matching objects to pictures and pictures to objects.

Following each session, the therapist working with the child completes a progress note that indicates what was done (e.g., which goals were addressed and for how long; data), how the child responded to intervention (assessment), and what is recommended. Progress notes facilitate communication among everyone working with the child, including the child's parents, who can review progress notes at any time.

Jesi did very well learning important basic skills using a DTI approach. Over the first few months, her parents were apprehensive about her slow progress, but once Jesi adjusted to therapy and began enjoying working with the therapists, her skills really took off.

After a year of DTI intervention, Jesi is clearly a different little girl. She is much less agitated and apprehensive than at the beginning of the intervention. When Jesi and her parents visited their family in Texas at about the 1-year point, her grandparents and aunts and uncles were flabbergasted at how much her behavior has improved. She has learned an array of new actions by video modeling, and her verbal greeting and expressive labeling have markedly improved. She's better at saying, "Bye" than "Hi," but she's making solid progress. Sometimes she uses "Bye" as a means of asking adults to leave if they are making demands she doesn't like, which we all find both clever and amusing. She is now using verbal requests to fulfill her needs and wants, so she is much less frustrated. Jesi is learning to tolerate a delay between making a request and an adult's complying with her request, which is helpful in avoiding meltdowns. Mom and Dad have applied behavioral intervention principles in teaching Jesi daily living skills, including dressing, toileting, and eating appropriately at meal times. They have taught her to wear headphones when confronted by loud noises that bother her, like the vacuum cleaner. The family's life together has greatly improved as Jesi has learned new skills and has fewer reasons to be upset or frightened by events beyond her control. All in all, Jesi has made impressive progress, but she has a long way to go before she is ready for school.

Family's Perspective: Jesi

"Every parent's ultimate goals for their child are. . . independence, personal success, and happiness. Those are some of ours, although we didn't realize they were [our goals] until Jesi was diagnosed with autism. We assumed success and independence would come naturally, but autism kind of took the "naturally" part away. But that didn't mean we couldn't try other things off the naturally beaten path.

After she was diagnosed, we were prodded to seek out speech and occupational therapy (OT), just like everyone else with the diagnosis. She received speech and OT for about 18 months and, in some respects, I would wager that her symptoms of autism had worsened. Her echolalia had increased, and she was just a walking [firestorm of] frustration toward adults and the world that they ran. The last 4 or 5 months of those 18, we added feeding therapy to help her learn to enjoy a larger variety of foods.

In feeding [therapy], I liked the idea that they started with something she liked, like M&Ms, and dipped them. . . in pudding, a texture she detests, but over time she enjoyed it. From that it went to applesauce, then apples, then pears, [and so forth]. It was building from something small, fun, and basic. The [feeding] therapist told me it was a lot like ABA therapy. I had never heard of ABA, but decided if it worked for food, why not teach her skills in a similar teaching pattern for other aptitudes that needed work? It's simple, Jesi found it predictable, and she also found success in the way of rewards to keep her motivated and trying.

So that's what started my research of ABA. The more I researched, the more I fell in love with not only the theory of it, but its modern-day practice. Then it came down to finding places that offered the highest intensity (in hours) where we could afford it. [Jesi]...was already behind, according to my reading, because most children who had higher rates of success got a hold of this therapy a lot sooner than we did. Speech therapy and occupational therapy alone clearly made no sense to Jesi. . . . and she didn't wear the look of happiness that comes from success and achievement. It got to where I was canceling [appointments] just to avoid an inevitable meltdown or irritability that would last for days or until the day before the next session. . . and she only had it twice a week. . . .I don't disagree with speech and occupational therapy—I see their uses and applications—but it was as though there were huge links in the chain missing that would have enabled her to make gains with them . . .ABA fills in those links that are missing.

I was very excited to start with the Minnesota Early Autism Project. At first, my hopes and expectations were more [based on]. . . .Jesi than the therapy. I knew if she could just latch on to the rhythm of therapy-reward-happiness-therapy-reward-happiness. . . she could do everything they were going to ask of her. It's the most basic steps of "learning how to learn." There were times that felt slower than others, but thank goodness for the meticulous graphs and excellent data collection so you can actually see the progress when it just looks stagnant to an optimistic (but concerned) mother. I can't remember how many times we've had to tell family on the phone, "she's coming along," wanting to give specific updates in the beginning, but it would be too hard to explain or for them to understand. Now, I can say she does this and this and this, and blew right through these goals. . . Like any great work, it doesn't happen fast and patience is essential.

I was surprised by a couple things. You'll hear a million times, "This works for my kid, it'll work on yours" [from parents whose kids are involved in other therapies]. Here [at Minnesota Early Autism Project], it's so personal and tailored to Jesi that there's really no room for failure. Jesi has a senior behavior therapist (SBT) who oversees the masterful "weaving" of the tapestry of skills Jesi needs and the proper ways that Jesi will need those skills taught. When something isn't working for Jesi, her SBT is on it before Jesi [experiences]. . . failure and frustration. Usually it's a minor tweak in the way something is presented, but other times it's something that only she will see and have us all correct to help Jesi become successful. . . I was not expecting that, and that's huge to us; we love our SBT and are always impressed with her talent and intuition.

I was also surprised with the therapists' demeanor. I had read books by parents whose children went through behavioral therapy. The parents spoke fondly of the therapist's work, not necessarily of the person, and that it was hard to watch their child struggle with the beginning process. It couldn't have been more different for me. I loved the work that these women [behavior therapists] put in; I was impressed by how unique their styles are. They are all very personable and truly likeable, and in spite of their [differences in] style, their deliverance of therapy to Jesi is seamless. I knew with such continuity Jesi couldn't fail—it wouldn't confuse her. . . . So for me it was exciting to watch the beginning, because I didn't see confusion on Jesi's face—frustration at times, yes; confusion, no. I was expecting, by other parents' accounts, heartache in the beginning. It was all "up" for me, because I had seen failure on Jesi's face with other therapies, [and] it wasn't here.

So, this therapy means everything to us. I feel it is the [platform] on which the rest of her life will be built. All the roots of every blossom will be found in our time spent here. We'll [discover]. . . the happiness she gets from certain skills, the natural gifts she has with others, and where she will have to work harder on other abilities. I believe she has an immense capacity to learn if [therapy is conducted] the right way, and [Minnesota Early Autism Project] provides that way and expects *great achievements from her as well. The bar is never set too low for her here. . . That's absolutely priceless to me, because she'll only go as far as we expect her to."*

—*Terra, mother of 5½-year-old Jesi,*
diagnosed with Autism Spectrum Disorder

● ● ● ● ● ● ● ● ●

Like Jesi, Patrick, whom we discussed at the beginning of the chapter, was a slow starter. Figure 7.10 summarizes Patrick's progress over the past 6 months on several of the skills it was determined were necessary for him to acquire.

SUMMARY

Children with little or no language attainment, very short attention span, lack of social interest, and substantial competing nonfunctional repetitive behavior are often good candidates for a DTI approach. They usually exhibit insufficient appropriate

Progress Study

Child's name: __Patrick_____ Date of birth: __10/26/06_____

Study date: __5/09_____

Goal	Baseline and progress data	Current status
Imitation with and without objects	Baseline zero (Date:____) 5 multiple actions (5/09)	Imitating 35 single and multiple actions Continue fine motor and oral imitation
Responding to instructions	Baseline zero (5/09)	9 mastered (8/09)
Eye contact when making requests	Baseline 15% (6/09)	85% (2/10)
Receptive identification	Baseline zero to 2 (3/09) Increased to 13 (Date___)	Mastered 8 receptive identifications in random order
Independent task completion	Baseline played independently with 4 toys (2/09)	Plays independently with 13 toys
Vocal imitation	Baseline zero (9/09)	Imitates 10 sounds reliably; produces a large number of single words including requests and labeling

Figure 7.10. Progress study for Patrick. Like Jesi, Patrick had a slow start but began making more rapid gains over the course of his first year of intervention. After one year he was saying single words, exhibiting eye contact when making requests, and playing independently with a wider array of toys.

adaptive behavior for using a naturalistic or Incidental Teaching approach based on following a child's lead. The DTI strategy is rooted in basic ABA learning theory principles. Periodic criterion-referenced testing, such as the VB-MAPP or ABLLS-R, as well as ongoing progress measurements of key outcome measures (e.g., percentage correct per opportunity, absolute number of responses per session) can be performed to gauge a child's skill acquisition. DTI has proven highly effective for at least half of the children with autism receiving such services, with the other half improving as well but often exhibiting less dramatic gains. Many parents are able to incorporate DTI procedures into normal daily routines, such as during meal times, bathing, or bedtime.

REFERENCES

Bond, L. (1996). Norm- and criterion-referenced testing. ERIC/AE Digest. *ERIC Educational Reports*. Educational Resources Information Center of the U.S. Department of Education. (ERIC Document Reprodouction Service No. ED402327)

Cooper, J.O., Heron, T.E., & Heward, W.L. (2007). *Applied behavior analysis* (2nd ed.). Upper Saddle River, NJ: Pearson.

Dickson, C.A., Wang, S.S., Lombard, K.M., & Dube, W.V. (2006). Overselective stimulus control in residential school students with intellectual disabilities. *Research in Developmental Disabilities, 27*(6), 618–631.

Ferster, C.B. (1953). The free operant in the analysis of behavior. *Psychological Bulletin, 50*(4), 263–274.

Lovaas, O.I. (1967). A behavior therapy approach to the treatment of childhood schizophrenia. *Minnesota Symposia on Child Psychology, 1,* 108–159.

Lovaas, O.I., Koegel, R.L., Simmons, J.Q., & Long, J. (1973). Some generalization and follow-up measures on autistic children in behavior therapy. *Journal of Applied Behavior Analysis, 6,* 131–166.

Maurice, C. (Ed.). (1996). *Behavioral intervention for young children with autism*. Austin, TX: Pro-Ed.

Montgomery, L.M. (1908). *Anne of Green Gables* [Electronic version]. Retrieved April 9, 2010, from http://www.gutenberg.org/etext/45

Partington, J.W. (2007). *Assessment of basic language and learning skills-revised (ABLLS-R)*. Walnut Creek, CA: The Behavior Analysts.

Schreibman, L., Koegel, R.L., & Craig, M.S. (1977). Reducing stimulus overselectivity in autistic children. *Journal of Abnormal Child Psychology, 5*(4), 425–436.

Smith, T., Groen, A., & Wynn, J. (2000). Randomized trial of intensive early intervention for children with pervasive developmental disorder. *American Journal on Mental Retardation, 105,* 269–285.

Sparrow, S.S., Cicchetti, D.V., & Balla, D.A. (2005). *Vineland Adaptive Behavior Scales–II (VABS-II)* (2nd ed.). Bloomington, MN: AGS Publishing/Pearson Assessments.

Sundberg, M. (2008). *Verbal Behavior Milestones Assessment and Placement Program*. Concord, CAA: Advancement of Verbal Behavior Press.

Sundberg, M.L. (2008). *Verbal behavior milestones assessment and placement program (VB-MAPP)*. Concord, CA: Advancements in Verbal Behavior Press.

Syrus, P. (1894). Maxim 439. In R. Bickford-Smith, Ed., *Sententiae* [Electronic version]. Retrieved April 7, 2010, from http://www.archive.org/details/publiliisyrisen00blicgoog

Wechsler, D. (2002). *Wechsler Preschool and Primary Scale of Intelligence* (WPPSI) (3rd ed.). Bloomington, MN: Pearson Assessments.

8

Incidental Interventions for Children with Moderate Autism Symptoms and Typical Intellectual Functioning

with Amy Bohannan

Question: "You prefer to be natural?"
Reply: "Sometimes. But it is such a very difficult pose to keep up."

—Oscar Wilde, *An Ideal Husband* (1912/2009)

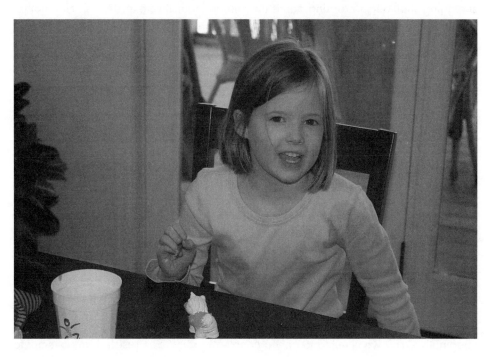

• • • • • • • • • •

INTRODUCTION: LILLY

Lilly was 4½ years old when she and her parents first visited our clinic to determine whether she might profit from EIBI therapy for children with ASDs. She had shoulder-length, tawny brown hair; brown eyes; and an attentive, engaging facial expression. Lilly's movements were animated and a bit theatrical. Her parents had first become concerned about her development when at age 2 she spoke only a few words and had developed rigid ways of doing things. She had tantrums when there was a change from what she expected. She screamed and resisted brushing her hair or teeth. Lilly had been evaluated by her local school district and found to qualify for educational services in the autism spectrum category. Her pediatrician diagnosed her with Asperger syndrome. Lilly had been receiving private speech and occupational therapy services, attending early childhood special education classes 6 hours per week, and receiving 1 hour per week of skills training at an autism specialty clinic. Lilly's parents felt she wasn't making adequate progress. Their main concerns were her inability to self-soothe and emotionally regulate and her excessive rigidity and meltdowns. They sought our help in improving her ability to interact socially with family members and peers.

Throughout her clinic visit, Lilly was very actively engaged, talking almost non-stop, at times in a sing-song voice. Her vocabulary seemed precocious, including using words like *exceptional* and *adventures* to describe toy play with toy animals and their activities. She was particularly absorbed with a toy merry-go-round and the characters associated with it. Lilly comfortably talked with a therapist seated alongside her on the floor. Lilly's questions and comments seemed perfunctory. After asking the therapist a question, she didn't wait for the therapist's reply or ignored it, continuing with her play as though she hadn't heard the therapist's response. She did not use gestures or seem to respond to others' gestures or body language (e.g., shrugging shoulders or turning palms up with an inquisitive expression). Her mother reported that Lilly was interested in other children but didn't seem to know how to initiate or maintain interactive play. She had limited tolerance for turn-taking or for losing during games. Lilly became upset when her younger brother, Charlie, cried, but only because she disliked the sound of crying. She became angry with him if he wouldn't stop. Although she enjoyed affection from her parents, she demonstrated little empathy toward others.

Lilly did not begin to use speech functionally until she was 2½ years old. Then her speech ability seemed to explode. Within a few months she was talking fluently and appeared to understand most things that adults said to her, but her expressive communication was often tangential and involved unusual, made-up words. Even when she knew the correct word for a situation, she often made up her own word, sometimes based on a property of the person or thing in question. For example, Lilly's teacher was called "Ms. Wendy" by the other students, but Lilly called her "Ms. Curly" because her hair was curly. She named her stuffed animals by their size or color, such as Small (her most preferred stuffed dog) or Blackie (not so unusual). When her brother received a toy dinosaur as a holiday present, she said, "It's a tiny, whiney, slimy, diney." When Lilly liked people, such as her senior behavior therapist, and thought they were funny, she said such things as "Ms. Amy, you're silly, willy, quilly," which she accompanied with a silly dance.

Lilly seemed to enjoy make-believe play, but her mother reported that her imaginative play was limited to only a couple of topics. She resisted any attempt to introduce a new topic. Lilly often narrated or commented on her imaginative play, which is common for typical children her age but infrequent with children on the autism spectrum. Lilly had no unusual movements, such as twirling in circles or flicking her fingers, nor did she stare at moving objects such as ceiling fans or flickering lights as do some children on the autism spectrum. Lilly's mother said Lilly had several fixed daily routines, such as bedtime preparation, which must be followed precisely or she would have a meltdown. Occasionally during meltdowns she scratched her face and body with her fingernails.

Lilly's mother completed a Gilliam Autism Rating Scale-2 (Gilliam, 2006), yielding an Autism Index Score in the "Possible Autism" range, and we completed a Childhood Autism Rating Scale (CARS; Schopler, Van Bourgondien, Wellman, & Love, 2010) based on observations and an interview with her mother, yielding a total CARS score of 30, which is at the lower end of the mildly to moderately autistic range. Earlier in the year, the school district had conducted an Autism Diagnostic Observation Schedule Module I (Lord, Rutter, DiLavore, & Risi, 1989). Her total score was well above the cutoff for autism (in the range often associated with Autistic Disorder).

When Lilly was seen in our clinic, she was diagnosed with Asperger Disorder. Our clinical team, including her parents, concluded that it was likely she would profit from a naturalistic EIBI therapy program built around her typical daily activities and routines. Therapy was initiated a little over a year prior to the time of this writing. Lilly's parents, Cindy and Doug, are both very bright and have postgraduate educational backgrounds. They had read a good deal about autism interventions and talked with other parents of children on the autism spectrum. They had heard some negative things about ABA, which they equated with UCLA Young Autism Project DTI. They were unfamiliar with naturalistic behavioral autism intervention and seemed uncertain about our staff member's ability to really get to know Lilly and them sufficiently in order to tailor an intervention strategy that was both effective and would fit well within their family. They decided to give it a try. A year later, they concluded that our joint efforts have worked well for Lilly and them.

When Lilly's entry characteristics were rated using the Autism Intervention Responsiveness Scale (AIRS™; Figure 8.1) she obtained an average rating of 2.55, suggesting she would be a strong candidate for Incidental Intervention. Lilly's main challenges were in difficulty expressing social interest, insistence on sameness, and narrow interests and social anxiety—with her very narrow interests posing the most significant intervention issues.

● ● ● ● ● ● ● ● ● ●

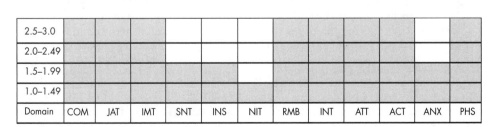

2.5–3.0												
2.0–2.49												
1.5–1.99												
1.0–1.49												
Domain	COM	JAT	IMT	SNT	INS	NIT	RMB	INT	ATT	ACT	ANX	PHS

Figure 8.1. Lilly's baseline Autism Intervention Responsiveness Scale (AIRS™) Profile (*Key:* COM, Communication; JAT, Joint Attention; IMT, Imitation; SNT, Social Interest; INS, Insistence on Sameness; NIT, Narrow Interests, RMB, Repetitive Motor Behavior; INT, Intellectual Ability; ATT, Attention; ACT, Activity; ANX, Anxiety/Fearfulness; PHS, Physical Features)

THERAPY PRINCIPLES AND ASSUMPTIONS

Although principles of naturalistic or incidental behavioral intervention involve the same stimulus control and reinforcement concepts as those in more structured behavioral intervention, there are significant differences. Those differences derive from early work in Incidental Language Learning and Milieu Language Teaching, which is closely related to Pivotal Response Training.

Roots in Incidental Language Learning

Naturalistic behavioral intervention for children with autism emerged from incidental teaching and milieu language intervention developed in the 1960s and 1970s. Incidental teaching (Hart & Risley, 1975) involves the use of normally occurring situations and the child's interest to facilitate learning. Originally, the strategy was focused on language learning, but later it was extended to include social skills as well (Koegel & Frea, 1993; McGee, Almeida, Sulzer-Azaroff, & Feldman, 1992). In incidental teaching, the therapist or caregiver takes advantage of naturally occurring daily situations in which to provide learning opportunities for the child. The situation or activity is child-selected (Hart & Risley, 1975), with the caregiver following the child's lead or interest. Incidental teaching strategies are ABA-based, designed to maximize reinforcement and facilitate generalization (Warren & Gazdag, 1990; Warren & Kaiser, 1986).

Peterson (2004) provided an excellent review of naturalistic language interventions. Elements of his discussion are incorporated in the following section. Kaiser defined milieu language teaching as "a naturalistic, conversation-based teaching procedure in which the child's interest in the environment is used as a basis for eliciting elaborated child communicative responses" (1993, p. 77). Naturalistic teaching approaches have been described as "structured approaches that use the natural routines and activities in natural environments as the teaching context" (Noonan & McCormick, 1993, p. 22). These "in-setting" natural environments may be the child's home, classroom, day care, or community settings. Once a teacher or caregiver identifies naturally occurring situations in which a child expresses interest, she or he uses a series of graduated prompts to encourage the child's responses (Hart & Risley, 1975; McGee, Krantz, & McClannahan, 1985).

Mand-Model

In ABA parlance, a request is called a *mand*. The teacher or therapist observes the object of the child's interest (e.g., a ball on a shelf out of reach) and models the appropriate spoken descriptor (e.g., "ball"). If the child makes the correct response (e.g., "ball"), the teacher or caregiver praises the child and gives him or her the item with which to play.

Next, the therapist or parent mands (requests) a response from the child (e.g., "Tell me what you want"). If the child makes an incorrect response (e.g., "bus" instead of "ball"), the teacher or caregiver models the correct response (e.g., "Say ball"). In teaching social skills, a similar strategy applies. For example, the therapist notes that the child especially enjoys playing the board game Candyland. The therapist takes a turn jumping her board piece and then says, "What do you want?" and looks at the child. The child responds by saying, "My turn." The therapist points to the spinner on the board and says, "Okay, your turn!"

In the mand-model procedure, the therapist or caregiver controls the number and frequency of opportunities for the child to verbally or socially interact (Rogers-Warren

& Warren, 1980). This procedure may be especially useful for children with very limited spontaneous initiation (Warren, McQuarter, & Rogers-Warren, 1984). Incidental teaching is dependent upon the child's spontaneous initiations rather than the therapist or teacher's prompts, and therefore requires greater early language and social skills, which consequently limits its use for prelinguistic or other nonspeaking children.

Time-Delay

Another extension of incidental teaching is the time-delay prompt procedure. *Time-delay* refers to nonvocal cues for spoken language (Halle, Baer, & Spradlin, 1981, p. 390). In the time-delay procedure, the parent, teacher, or therapist identifies a situation in which the child wants access to something or needs assistance and waits for the child to make a response—hence the *delay*. If the child does not respond (Child: "ball" or "help"), another delay is instituted. Often if the therapist is patient, the child will make an approximation of the correct response (e.g., "ba-"). If this second delay does not produce an appropriate child response, the caregiver or teacher switches to the mand-model procedure. The therapist asks, "What do you want?" and then after a short delay, the therapist models, "ball." The time-delay procedure is useful for teaching children to initiate verbal or social interactions (Noonan & McCormick, 1993).

Incidental teaching is largely spontaneous and guided by the child's interests. Knowing a child likes to play house, a parent says, "Let's play house," and sets a wooden toy house on the floor along with miniature family characters and items that might be used in a house, such as furniture, dishes, vacuum cleaner, and pet dog. From that point forward, the adult follows the child's lead. The child picks up a miniature adult male character and Mom says, "Who is that?" The child replies, "Daddy." "What should we do with Daddy?" Mom asks. The child places the man in the garage, and the mom asks, "Where is Daddy?" (requesting a preposition). The child responds by saying "in the garage." "Right!" the parent says. "He's *in* the garage." The specific skills taught within such scenarios are planned in advance based on the child's individualized treatment plan or IEP.

A risk associated with totally incidental naturalistic intervention strategy is that the child's spontaneous rate of relevant initiations may be so low that she or he doesn't receive enough practice with each skill, called *inadequate intensity*. A second issue is that incidental teaching or therapy requires exquisite sensitivity to *teachable opportunities specifically related to the child's educational or home therapy goals*. At times, less experienced staff members find themselves being drawn into a child's very interesting play activities that are, unfortunately, not necessarily relevant to the child's therapy or teaching goals. Effectively using an incidental therapy approach requires identifying points within the child's more commonly selected activities within which specific teaching goals can be readily embedded.

Occasional Discrete Trials to Teach New Skills

In Chapter 2, we noted that expression of the three core autism features (limited social skills, limited communication skills, and repetitive nonfunctional behavior) for a given child is often amplified by the degree of attention and anxiety problems. A capable child with some beginning language and social interest may nonetheless be highly distractible or apprehensive, and may resist spontaneously interacting with his or her teacher or therapist. It is not possible to predict with a great deal of accuracy whether a child will profit sufficiently from an incidental teaching approach based on their core autism symptoms and intellectual functioning alone. After an initial rapport-building period, a child with severe anxiety or ADHD symptoms often profits from a few weeks of DTI, employing materials with which the youngster has expressed special interest. As the child becomes increasingly able to focus her or his attention on the task at hand and the apprehensiveness gradually diminishes, it is often appropriate to make a transition to a mand-model procedure, described above, and then later to incidental teaching procedures involving more spontaneous child-selected activities. Once the child is successfully learning within the context of an incidental naturalistic teaching procedure, it is usually not necessary to use a DTI method unless the child suddenly begins having more attention or anxiety problems or she or he finds a new task too difficult.

Identify and Teach Broadly
Applicable Skills: Pivotal Response Treatment

PRT is an autism early intervention strategy based largely on principles of ABA, incorporating concepts drawn from incidental and milieu teaching (Hart & Risley, 1968; Kaiser, 1993; McGee, Krantz, & McClannahan, 1985). PRT was developed by Robert Koegel, Laura Schreibman, and colleagues (Koegel, Bimbela, & Schreibman, 1996; Pierce & Schreibman, 1995) and elaborated in collaboration with Lynn Kern Koegel (Koegel & Koegel, 2006). PRT was initially mainly a classroom intervention strategy in which behavioral interventions were ensconced within normal daily instructional activities and routines (Koegel & Frea, 1993). The same methods were encouraged at home as well, with parents assuming the "teacher" role. Over intervening years, PRT methods have been extended more broadly to a variety of community settings as well.

PRT is based on the premise that by teaching or strengthening certain *pivotal* skills, others will emerge automatically without being explicitly taught. Pivotal skills are behaviors that are central to a wide area of functioning. *Initiating interactions* and *requesting what the child wants* are pivotal skills that can be used in a wide variety of situations with various people and circumstances. PRT is a largely child-directed naturalistic intervention. Thus PRT is able to increase the generalization of new skills while increasing the motivation of children to perform the behaviors being taught to them. PRT works to increase motivation by including components such as child choice, turn-taking, reinforcing attempts, and interspersing maintenance tasks. PRT has been used to target language skills, play skills, and social behaviors in children with autism.

At Minnesota Early Autism Project, we incorporate elements of mand-modeling, incidental teaching, and PRT in our interventions for higher functioning children, for example, children who have Asperger syndrome or PDD-NOS. These interventions can be effective alone or in combination when tailored to the characteristics of the child.

Daily Routines-Based Intervention

Naturalistic interventions often work best if they are nested within normal daily routines at home or school rather than removing the child from those situations to conduct teaching or therapy (as in DTI or pull-out services in school). A *routine* at home or in school is an activity or period of the day during which specific activities (e.g., dressing, meal time, circle time) usually occur. Daily routines are not necessarily systematically planned; they may emerge in a particular way over time in the course of normal family life or school routines.

Routines-based interventions begin with characterizing the parent's satisfaction with a home routine or the teacher's judgment of the fit between the child and the classroom routine (McWilliam & Scott, 2001). Within daily routines, the therapy staff and parents or teachers and autism specialists identify periods during which specific therapy activities can be embedded without unduly altering the normal daily activity that would have occurred during that period (e.g., meal time at home, water table play at school). Periods during which parents or teachers indicate they are having specific challenges with the target child are often the focus of special attention (e.g., following parents' daily living activity requests, lining up for lunch).

Not all therapy or teaching activities need be part of an existing behavioral routine. In some cases, parents and therapy staff or teachers and specialist consultants may conclude it would be appropriate to insert a more carefully structured theme-based activity between existing daily routines (e.g., imaginative play centered around restaurant or doctor's office themes). It is especially helpful if those thematic activities can be linked to anticipated or recurring family events—such as a visit to the doctor's office or a family meal at a nearby restaurant—that provide opportunities for generalization.

Learning Is Initially Incremental and Later Progresses by Leaps and Bounds

Early in therapy, child learning is often plodding, and parents may feel their child is making little progress. After several weeks or months, their child's skills may suddenly improve for several weeks and then level off before finally taking off by leaps and bounds. An important part of naturalistic learning is called *learning to learn*. Initially children may be confused about the nature of the learning task. When a child is being taught to select vegetables from other food items for a restaurant thematic activity, she or he may initially think she or he is supposed to select only green things or the object on the left or the larger of several items. Once the child learns the nature of the discrimination task (e.g., any vegetable as opposed to nonvegetables), she or he readily learns to select items in a given category. With each new example of a type of discrimination (the next time it may be things with which one can play), children catch on more quickly, sometimes in only a few tries.

Capitalizing on the Child's Interests and Aptitudes

Most higher functioning children on the autism spectrum have several specific interests, such as weather, dinosaurs, specific animals (e.g., dogs or cats), types of vehicles, or story or video characters such as Thomas the Tank Engine. They may also have highly preferred activities, such as coloring with markers; printing letters, numbers or words; or sorting items into unique categories.

One of Lilly's ITP objectives was to *increase sharing her personal experiences* with her therapy staff, parents, and peers. The goal was to enable her to carry on a conversation about something that happened to her earlier in the day, or the previous day, with her family or others at a later time. Because Lilly was especially interested in animals, her therapists initially provided opportunities to select among several activities, one of which was playing with toy animals. She usually selected that activity. Sometimes the activity involved playing farm, other times taking the toy dog to the veterinarian, feeding the toy cat, and so on. Later, while talking with her mother, she was asked to report on what she did, using eye contact and appropriate gestures. Initially Lilly shared her experiences with her parents during approximately 30% of opportunities, called her *baseline*. After practicing with several highly preferred items and activities (e.g., drawing pictures of animals, creating story sequences with pictures, engaging in veterinarian pretend play) for 3 months, she shared her experiences with her parents approximately 90% of the time, obviously a substantial improvement. Subsequently, the procedure incorporated new activities that were not tailor-made to appeal to Lilly's interests, and she maintained the skill of sharing with her parents what she had done at school or on a community visit.

Invite the Child to Help Structure Learning Opportunities

Many naturalistic intervention activities can be planned jointly with the child. For children participating in thematic activities such as playing restaurant, the therapist or teacher begins by asking the child what he or she will need to play restaurant. This provides the opportunity for the child to develop vocabulary pertinent to various situations he or she will encounter in daily life. Complex, sometimes intimidating sets of activities are broken down into smaller, manageable routines. For example, when asked what they would need to play restaurant, 5-year-old Blake replied by saying they would need dishes, food items, and a table and chair. His therapist Ashley asked, "How will we know what food we can serve for lunch?" After a moment's thought Blake replied, "We need a menu." "Right," Ashley said. Blake decided he needed an apron if he was going to be a waiter in a restaurant, so his mother offered him a small one she no longer used. "I wonder what food is on the menu?" Ashley asked. Blake said, "I'll write *food* on the menu." Blake folded a piece of paper in half, printed the word *Menu* on the front with a red marker, and then began printing food items on the inside of the menu. He printed *orange juice* and *chicken fingers* on the menu. "Do you think your customers might like something else?" Ashley asked, requiring Blake to take the other person's perspective. "Corn and potatoes," Blake replied and printed them on the list. After several seconds he added, "ice cream." "How about broccoli?" Ashley asked. "No, people don't like broccoli," Blake replied, reflecting his dislike for the pungent vegetable.

Children are more highly motivated to participate in activities of their own making than those shaped entirely by their parents, teachers, or therapists. They are also more likely to remember words and concepts when their active responses are required than when these words and concepts are only spoken to them by others. "Now let's pretend you are the customer and I'm the waiter," Ashley continued. Blake took the seat by the table and looked up at Ashley. "What would you like for lunch, sir?" Ashley asked Blake. He thought for a moment and picked up the menu and selected two items. "Would you like anything with your chicken fingers?" Ashley asked.

"Catsup," Blake replied. Then Ashley modeled further perspective-taking, looking off in the distance away from Blake.

"Hmm, I wonder whether the customer would like something to drink," Ashley pretended she was thinking to herself. "Maybe I should ask him." By the time Ashley asked Blake what he wanted to drink, he had already thought about the answer and replied, "Orange juice." The next time Blake was the waiter, he followed her model and asked Ashley if she would like anything else with her lunch.

Depending on the activity, a child may be able to make or select nearly all of the materials required for a thematic play activity. Learning to determine what is missing to participate in an activity is a valuable lesson in itself. The same type of routine can be used with household chores, such as setting the table or assisting with meal preparation.

Overcoming and Managing Compulsive Rituals and Routines

With most children on the autism spectrum, compulsive symptoms and ritualistic behavior occur on and off during most waking hours. But for higher functioning children, repetitive compulsive routines are frequently situation-specific, such as getting ready to depart for school in the morning or preparing for bed in the evening. The child attempts to manage anxiety-producing transitions by developing rigid routines that reduce their anxiety and create a sense of control. For Lilly, each step of preparing for bed in the evening had to be followed in a very specific sequence, and if any step were skipped or for some reason not possible (e.g., if her regular pajamas were in the laundry), chaos would reign. She screamed and sobbed, bringing bedtime preparation to a standstill.

A combination of strategies can reduce rigidity, with patience and perseverance. Begin by discussing with the child the steps she believes must be followed. Next, a social story is prepared leading up to the step in which one item that is typically done in a particular way will be changed, for example the child's preferred bubble bath. Explain, "Tonight we are going to use a different bubble bath," and show the child the container of new bubble bath. If she cries or begins to tantrum, calmly repeat, "Tonight we're going to use this new bubble bath and it's going to be fun," and walk away from the child. Busy yourself with something else. As soon as the child begins calming down say, "What a big girl you are. Let's get ready for your bath." Give the child the new bubble bath to hold in her hand. Lift her into the tub and say, "Let's put in some bubbles," and help the child pour some of the new bubble bath in the tub. By giving the child some control over the change, it becomes less disturbing to her. Over the next 2 weeks, every other or every third night, change an additional aspect of the bedtime routine. Most children, like Lilly, become accustomed to an altered routine within a few weeks. Each time this strategy is used with another rigid routine, it becomes easier for the child as well as for the family or teacher in school. Eventually the child comes to trust that the adult will not expose him or her to a highly disturbing change.

Capitalizing on Social Interest and Overcoming Social Anxiety

When we see a bright, high-functioning child during a first visit to our clinic, one of our greatest concerns is whether he or she exhibits social interest. Does he look at his parents when they say something? Does she establish eye contact with me when I call her name? Does he show our therapist seated on the floor with him a toy he finds interesting? All of these observations bode very well for the child's making progress in developing social skills. Many higher functioning children are interested in being near and watching other children play, but typically do not know how to enter into play with their peers. That is also predictive of more rapid progress in learning social skills. Children who show little interest in other children are much more difficult to involve in learning interactive play and other social skills.

I have worked with parents who believed that, if they just plunked their child with autism down in the midst of a group of typical children in a preschool or on the playground, their son or daughter would "just get it" (i.e., know how to play with other children). In my experience, that is often a mistake. An anxious child with an ASD often panics in such a situation, descending into a meltdown that may last an hour or more. Alternatively, the child with autism retreats to a corner of the classroom or playground farthest away from his peers. That sets back progress in helping the child feel more socially comfortable and confident.

Children with substantial social anxiety can often learn to overcome much of their fear by gradual exposure to other children, beginning with one child at a time. By inviting a neighbor or friend's child over to the house to play, the child learns to be less fearful around other children. A child with an ASD may repeatedly mention another child's name when he arrives home from school, leading Mom to wonder about this child. When Mom checks with her son's teacher about who the child is, the teacher's voice sounds a note of alarm. She tells Mom that the youngster in question has problems in school and is not an ideal playmate for her son. It is common for youngsters with autism to find rambunctious, loud children most memorable, not because they like them, but because they are so overwhelming. Good playmates for children on the autism spectrum are calm, easygoing, and accepting. Often neurotypical preschool and kindergarten-age girls are more accepting and nurturing than same-age boys and make excellent playmates for both girls and boys on the autism spectrum. Preschool and kindergarten-age children are often forgiving of odd behavior as long as their new playmate is not aggressive. It is a good idea for adults to initially monitor play dates closely to make certain both children have positive experiences. By providing an adequate array of appropriate toys to avoid competition for specific toys and reminding the children to "play nicely," over time the child with an ASD will become less anxious around other children. Although typical children easily learn what to do from observing other children, those with ASDs generally do not. They need to be explicitly taught the prosocial and early social skills involved in initiating and maintaining social interactions.

Once play with a single child around the target child's chronological age has been successful, it may be time to add a third child. Sometimes that can be a sibling and other times a classmate from school. The three children can learn to take turns together, to comment on each other's craft projects, and to share snacks. Care must be taken to make certain the two typical children do not direct all of their interactions toward one another, effectively excluding the child with autism. Some older, higher functioning children can make use of Tony Attwood's "Emotional Toolbox" (Attwood, 2004; Chapter 5) skills when they become anxious, such as engaging in specific physical activities (e.g., jumping on a trampoline) or relaxing in a beanbag chair. Those with good verbal skills, like Lilly, can be taught self-talk skills, which can be helpful for some children (e.g., "I can be calm," "It's not a big deal").

Maintaining Intensity in Natural Settings

In Chapter 4 and in the previous section of the present chapter, we discussed the importance of maintaining adequate intervention intensity while conducting naturalistic interventions. While a teacher or behavior therapist is engaged with a child within a typical daily routine, such as mealtime or imaginative play, it is easy for the caregiver to lose sight of how frequently learning activities are directed toward achieving IEP or ITP goals. We generally recommend a supervising therapist work with the therapist and parents to create a concrete expectation regarding how many repetitions of specific learning opportunities are to occur per session.

● ● ● ● ● ● ● ● ●

Linda is a bright 6-year-old with Asperger Disorder who has narrow interests and does not recognize social cues indicating her playmates are bored. Her mother and therapists began by identifying contexts in which nonverbal social cues would be used. We embedded these into our activities. Second, they role-played with a variety of nonverbal cues to show why people use them and why it's important to change what we're doing. For example, therapists practiced looking away as Linda was continuing to talk, and they practiced asking Linda, "What's wrong?" or "What's up?" if she was unable to identify the nonverbal cue. After Linda could detect signs of boredom in therapists and her mother, the same skills were practiced with peers. Over time Linda learned to pay closer attention to social cues given by all conversational and play partners and to adjust her behavior accordingly.

Throughout these incidental-learning situations we encourage our therapy staff to track the number of repetitions of the specific learning activity about once per week using a tally counter attached to their waistband.

• • • • • • • • • •

Promoting Tolerance for Social Rejection

Most children with ASDs have difficulty initiating and maintaining social interactions with peers. Because their social overtures often lack nuance, children with ASDs are often rebuffed by peers who may prefer to play with other children. Higher functioning children are often sensitive to social rejection, and they either stop trying to interact or become upset and may have a meltdown. Our strategy is first to reduce the likelihood that our client or student's social overtures will be rejected, by teaching more effective skills. Then we teach the child something else to do rather than having an emotional outburst.

If a typically developing peer wants to join in play with other children, he or she often first observes what the other children are doing and then either comments on their play or may ask to join in. Children with ASDs often make the mistake of expecting the other children to stop what they are playing and switch to what the child with autism wants to play. This usually fails. We teach our children on the autism spectrum to begin by observing what their peers are doing and next to make a positive comment. For example, two boys are seated on the floor playing with cars. Barry, a 7-year-old child with Asperger Disorder, approaches, watches for 10 to 15 seconds, and then says, "Wow, that red car is really cool!" Often the other boys will look up and say, "Do you want to play?" If the boys do not respond this way, Barry was taught to say something like, "I have a blue car like yours. I'll show you." At this point the child with autism becomes part of the other two boys' play without further ado.

At times, despite the best efforts of a child with ASD, their peers may choose not to include them in their ongoing play. The target child can be taught several adaptive alternatives. The first is to look for another child or children with whom to play. Often this second attempt is successful. If not, we teach the child to engage in self-talk, first out loud and later subvocally: "It's okay if I don't play with them now. I'll play with them later." Or, "It's okay if I don't play with them now. I'll draw instead." The child is encouraged to have several back up alternative activities that she or he enjoys.

Generalizing to Natural Family and Community Settings

Most of the incidental teaching and thematic play activities used for naturalistic intervention are similar to activities in a child's real life with the family, such as going to the library, going shopping, visiting the dentist, and so forth. Once they meet mastery criteria within the incidental teaching or therapy context, most children are readily able to generalize to natural settings with their family. At times, additional sessions may be added in which the therapist and family visit community settings together to identify other problem areas. For example, Margy had difficulty going shopping without insisting on having specific items from the store, such as toiletries, and if she didn't get them she had an emotional outburst. A behavioral contracting procedure was used in which

Margy was promised one small item from the toiletry section if she did not whine or otherwise attempt to secure other toiletry items. If she whined or complained, no toiletries were purchased that shopping trip. If she didn't whine or complain, after all other shopping had been completed, Margy and her mother visited the toiletries and she selected one small item.

ROOTS IN APPLIED BEHAVIOR ANALYSIS PRINCIPLES

As with earlier interventions noted in this book, naturalistic interventions are rooted in principles of ABA but draw upon developmental concepts as well. They employ methods developed as components of milieu language intervention, incidental teaching, and PRT, which were outgrowths of behavior analysis methods. Although trial-by-trial data are often not maintained with naturalistic interventions, the method is nonetheless data intensive. Typically, probe periods are interspersed periodically during sessions in which data are collected to determine whether the intervention is effective.

Setting: Venues Throughout the Home, School, and Other Community Sites

The settings in which intervention is conducted are defined largely by the places in which the child typically participates in her or his daily routines. At home, generally no one room is designated as the therapy room, though that may at times be helpful early in therapy. Therapy or learning sessions are not done at a table in a single location. In school, intervention is often done in learning stations or centers throughout the classroom, in the gym or on the playground, in the lunchroom, library, or music room.

Supplies

Although all materials are situated within reach on or near the table or floor when conducting DTI services, usually parents designate specific storage cabinets in rooms throughout the house where different therapy materials are kept, depending on the activity (e.g., board games, arts and crafts supplies, dress-up costumes). As much as possible, children are invited to participate in getting materials ready for therapy sessions by identifying what supplies are needed and retrieving them from their storage locations. Some supplies such as stickers, score sheets, or other tangible or consumable reinforcers are kept in a separate "adults only" locked cabinet.

Assessment

Figure 8.2 shows Lilly's baseline skills and 1-year performance on the ABLLS-R (Partington, 2007). The upper chart shows her baseline performance on cooperation, visual skills, receptive language, imitation, vocal imitation, requests, and labeling, while the lower charts show Lilly's baseline and 1-year performance on syntax and grammar, play and leisure skills, social interaction skills, and performance in group instruction situations. The last four charts of skills that are used in school settings were not completed. Although Lilly performed well on most basic skills, she exhibited significant deficits in social skills and interactive play. After 1 year, nearly all of those deficits had been overcome.

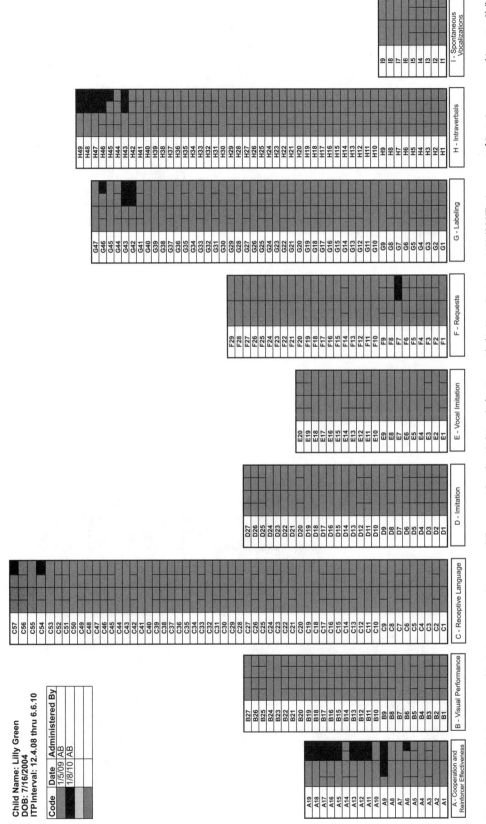

Figure 8.2. Lilly's Assessment of Basic Language and Learning Skills scores at baseline (light) and after 1 year (dark). (From Partington, J.W. (2007). *Assessment of Basic Language and Learning Skills-Revised (ABLLS-R)*. Walnut Creek, CA: The Behavior Analysts, Inc.; adapted by permission.)

(continued)

Figure 8.2. *(continued)*

Child Name: Lilly Green
DOB: 7/16/ 2004
ITP Interval: 12/4/08 through 6.6.10

Code	Date	Administered By
	1/5/09	AB
	1/8/10	AB

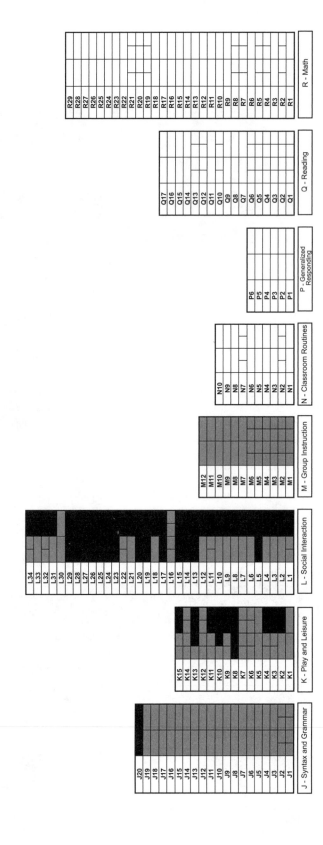

Figure 8.3, provided by Dr. Mark Sundberg, shows baseline skill levels for a high functioning child, Duval, whose abilities are similar to Lilly's. Note that compared with the VB-MAPP example in Chapter 7 for a child receiving DTI, Duval scores near the ceiling on all of the Level 1 skills expected of a birth to 18-month-old child, and even displays many Level 2 skills of an 18- to 30-month-old child and some of those of a 30- to 48-month-old child (Level 3; Sundberg, 2008).

● ● ● ● ● ● ● ● ●

BEGINNING THERAPY

Initially, Lilly insisted on having control over virtually all activities that involved her in any way. When therapists first entered her home and began placing any demands on her, no matter how small, severe power struggles ensued. Starting

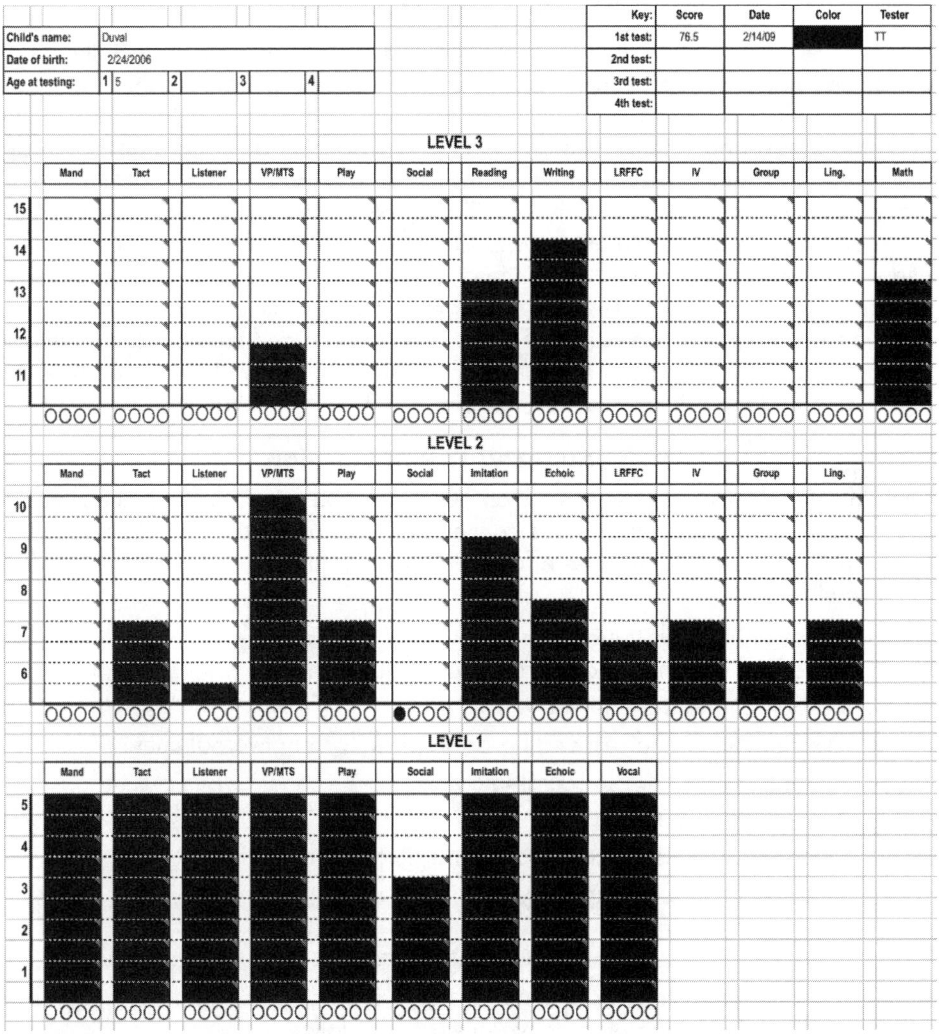

Figure 8.3. Duval's Verbal Behavior Milestones Assessment and Placement Program results, provided by Dr. Mark Sundberg, illustrating baseline test results for a child of skills similar to those of Lilly. (From http://www.marksundberg.com; reprinted by permission.)

intervention required making it possible for Lilly to tolerate having less control. An initial schedule was established of activities of specific interest to Lilly, such as animal-related activities. Lilly was encouraged to select the first three or four activities and then the therapist chose one activity. The number of Lilly's choices was gradually reduced until the therapist could pick several activities before Lilly had her choice of what to do, always giving Lilly some choices within those activities. For example, if the therapist decided the next activity involved playing a game, she gave Lilly the choice between two games. Over time, Lilly tolerated having less control without descending into screaming and crying. Once therapy staff members were able to reduce Lilly's rigidity and need for control of all activities, it was possible to address other therapy objectives.

Lilly is very bright and obviously more capable than the way she functioned at baseline, but her severe, compulsive need for control limited her development. Overcoming her need for control was a first priority.

Lilly at Baseline

Lilly was very rigid in her daily routines. She had narrow interests, especially in animals, and had low tolerance for playing with any toys or games other than animals. She felt a need to determine what and how she wanted to play and gave each toy a novel name. Her need for control extended to arts and crafts, as well. Lilly became extremely frustrated when participating in an art or craft activity if she made mistakes and it was "not perfect." If she colored out of the lines during a coloring activity, she cried, screamed, and ripped her paper. She displayed very limited eye contact during social interactions. Lilly was noncompliant or unresponsive to most adult requests directed to her without a highly motivating outcome for her (e.g., access to her favorite animal, Small). Lilly, parents, and therapy staff often got into power struggles over her noncompliance. Lilly would say "I know you have to leave soon and your time is up, so I'm going to sit here until you leave."

Individualized Treatment Plan

Lilly's initial individualized treatment plan goals were based on her baseline ABLLS-R assessment, interviews with parents concerning their priorities, and staff observations. The first 8 of 29 objectives addressed over her first year of therapy included the following:
  1. Increased verbal requesting
  2. Increased correct responding to "WH" questions
  3. Responding to multiple-step instructions
  4. Discriminating and responding appropriately to nonverbal cues
  5. Increased initiations in social interactions
  6. Turn-taking without tantrums
  7. Decreased obsessive-compulsive and ritualistic behaviors
  8. Increased tolerance for delay

Sample Outcome

Of the 29 objectives established as part of Lilly's individualized treatment plan, she mastered all goals within a year. Several examples follow.

Reading Nonverbal Cues: Lilly was initially unable to distinguish nonverbal social cues, such as frowns, shrugging shoulders, or looking bored. A program was developed to address this deficit. Figure 8.4 graphically shows Lilly's

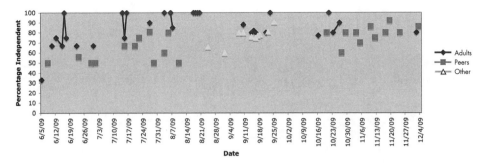

Figure 8.4. Lilly's acquisition of skills in reading and responding appropriately to nonverbal cues. Diamonds show responding to adult cues, squares show results for responding to same-age peers' nonverbal cues, and triangles show results for unfamiliar people.

learning of nonverbal social cues. Diamonds are data for correctly recognizing adult cues and squares signify recognizing nonverbal cues provided by same-age peers. Triangles represent cues provided by others, such as neighbors or strangers.

Joining in Play: Lilly was often bossy and found it difficult to enter into other children's play without dominating the choice of activities and how the activities were to be carried out. This led other children to lose interest or to be unwilling to play with her. In Figure 8.5, accurately observing and noting what peers are playing and doing is shown in diamonds. Commenting on what peers are doing, such as "Hey, that's a cool baby doll!" is shown in squares. Successfully joining into peers' play is shown in triangles.

Empathy Toward Others: Lilly had little understanding of others' emotions and showed little or no empathy toward people, though she did exhibit concern about her toy animals' feelings. Addressing this skill required two steps. First, Lilly learned to discriminate others' feelings and was able to explain that they were the same as her feelings when she was happy, sad, angry, and so forth. The next step involved teaching her to express supportive feelings toward others, beginning with her little brother, Charlie, then family members, and finally peers. In Figure 8.6, progress in identifying feelings and expressing empathy in therapist-contrived situations is shown in squares, and accuracy of

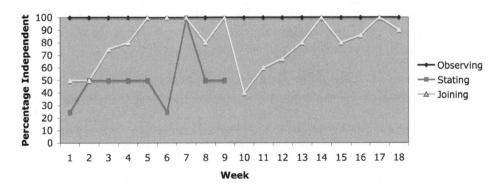

Figure 8.5. Lilly's learning to enter into ongoing peer play by observing (diamonds) and commenting (squares) on the peer's play and then joining (triangles).

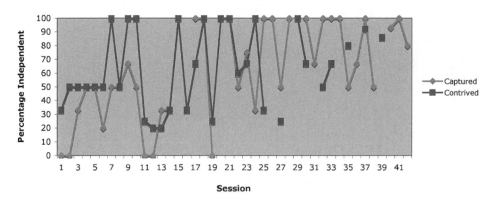

Figure 8.6. Graphic representation of Lilly's progress in learning to feel and express empathy toward others. Simulations are shown in squares and spontaneously captured natural events are shown in diamonds.

doing so in naturally occurring spontaneous situations is shown in diamonds. The graph in Figure 8.6 is quite variable, because from day to day the total number of empathy opportunities was small, but the overall trend is clear.

Sharing Experiences: At baseline, Lilly seldom told her parents or other adults about interesting things that had happened to her earlier in the day, such as at camp or in school. She was taught how to remember interesting events. Initially, therapists focused on Lilly's ability to answer more complex "WH" questions and the concepts of *yesterday, today,* and *tomorrow.* Next Lilly was sent on errands that required following at least three-step instructions. When she returned, she was asked questions regarding her tasks (e.g., "Where did you go?" "What did you do?" "Who did you see?"). Lilly already had substantial baseline knowledge of places and events and displayed a precocious vocabulary, so it was unnecessary to teach her new words. Once she was reporting accurately on things that happened today and yesterday and were going to happen tomorrow, we expanded it to questions such as "What did you do with Mama Green on Saturday?" Lilly's parents and nanny followed through and expressed genuine interest in her responses. Lilly seemed to be aware of her family's interest in her reports and began adding more details to her descriptions, on her own. That made it possible to gradually fade out most of the adult questions as Lilly became more interested in sharing her experiences with others and became interested in others' experiences. Her progress in reporting specific items was more rapid, shown in squares in Figure 8.7, but she also grew progressively more accurate in describing her experiences, for example, things that were the most fun (diamonds).

Lilly After One Year of Therapy

Lilly was evaluated at a multidisciplinary pediatric autism clinic after 1 year of therapy. Her verbal intelligence was 114 and performance IQ was 100, yielding a full-scale IQ of 104, in the average range. Her vocabulary test score was in the superior range. Her receptive and expressive language test scores were in the superior range. Lilly's VABS-II composite score was 101, or average. Her ADOS on Module 3 (advanced) was in the low spectrum range, but not in the Autistic Disorder range. She retained a diagnosis of Asperger Disorder.

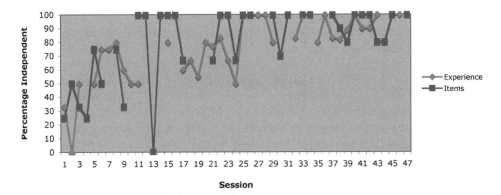

Figure 8.7.   Lilly's incidental learning of sharing her experiences with parents and therapists. She found it easier to recall and report specific things (items) that occurred than events requiring reporting her own reactions to those things.

Lilly has made great interpersonal strides. She now plays interactively with peers, is able to take turns, and tolerates losing. Now, when her brother cries, she tries to help him or seeks her parent's assistance for him. She expresses concern about her parents' feelings. She now recognizes emotions from people's facial expressions and gestures and has begun to learn to act accordingly by hugging or offering to help or joining in their pleasure. She is participating in regular play dates with girls her age. Though she continues to be a bit bossy and impatient at times, she and her friends generally get along well and enjoy their time together. Last summer Lilly attended a 1-month outdoor nature camp, where she was able to find a variety of animals interesting in addition to dogs, with which she was preoccupied in the beginning. Nine months after therapy outset, Lilly began spending half days in a regular education classroom in a science magnet school and is doing well both academically and socially. She has had no behavioral challenges in school.

Lilly is able to tolerate variations in her daily routines without meltdowns. Her main persistent challenge is perfectionism. Her parents developed a verbal strategy for helping Lilly decide whether it was worth becoming upset if something happened (including her own performance) that wasn't to her satisfaction. When she appeared to be getting upset, they would ask Lilly, "Is it a big deal or a little deal?" They taught her that most things were a "little deal" and not worth getting upset about. "Big deals" were difficult situations, such as when Grandma had to go to the hospital or when their pet dog ran away, and in those cases it was all right to become upset. The strategy helped Lilly avoid turning minor daily events into catastrophes.

Family's Perspective: Lilly

Like most parents being told for the first time that something might be amiss with their child from an outsider—in this case, our daughter Lilly's Montessori teacher— we were uncertain of where to turn first. Since the early childhood special education department within our school district where we live offered minimally invasive help and assessments, we started with them. Once they confirmed something was amiss and loosely assigned that "something" a name—autism spectrum disorder— the options of where to run to first (not walk!) were truly overwhelming.

With an "educational label" of simply "ASD" from the school district in hand, the next thing we believed we needed was a clear and definitive medical diagnosis.

That is, what, exactly, does Lilly have? We wanted a name, a specific name. Then, after poring over books and web sites, talking with other parents, and turning to professional resources, we quickly realized that the official label given was less important than honing in on Lilly's specific impairments and beginning to address those impairments—and as soon as possible. Adjusting our mind-set in this way saved us invaluable time and allowed us to begin the task of selecting and starting treatments sooner rather than later.

The list of potential treatments was overwhelming and intimidating. The choices included occupational therapy, speech therapy, special education services through our school district, biomedical therapies (including but not limited to drug interventions and dietary approaches such as a gluten-free and casein-free diet and/or vitamin supplementation), ABA, ABA/VB [ABA plus Verbal Behavior intervention], RDI [Relationship Development Intervention], DIR/Floortime, XYZ, LMNOP!

During one appointment with Lilly's pediatrician, who specializes in mental health, we were given one of the more salient pieces of advice we received on the numerous treatment options: "Give 'em all a try. Get Lilly as much help as you can and from as many angles as you can. Although there will be some crossover with these interventions, many of these services will complement each other. My experience has been that all interventions work at least some for most kiddos."

We proceeded in that direction; that is, we started all of the services we could get our hands on, all at the same time. Our approach meant that the OT would have to accept and incorporate the ABA and RDI work we were doing, the ABA behavioral therapists (BTs) would have to do the same with the OT and RDI goals that we had, and ditto for the RDI-folk with regard to our ABA and OT initiatives. And we would have to disregard any disapproving looks by them all. So be it.

It turns out that the providers we employed—some were chosen by luck and others by investigative skills—were and are progressive and inclusive of most, if not all, ASD interventions. And because of that, it's been easy to coordinate their efforts as it relates to Lilly's impairments and needs.

Noteworthy in her treatment plan is the behavioral intervention treatment that she receives from her ABA provider, Minnesota Early Autism Project (MEAP). We were initially skeptical and apprehensive of this intensive approach (20+ hours per week). How can strangers come into our home and make changes to Lilly's behavior when we have been unable to do so as her parents for the last 2 years? Well, they have and they are. MEAP's BTs are skilled and well-trained; of equal importance, they accept, understand, and seem to genuinely enjoy helping Lilly and our family. Simply put, ABA intervention through MEAP has been life changing for us. This intervention is being complemented by occupational therapy, speech therapy, and social skills training.

Lilly has now been receiving services—of all kinds—for 1 year. We've been astonished at the changes in Lilly. Specifically, is Lilly more compliant? Yes. Is she more flexible? Yes. Is she less controlling? Yes. Is she more willing to accept mistakes (of herself and others)? Yes. Does she have more social skills? Yes. More important than all of those individual components, is Lilly a happier little girl, one who more freely hugs her family, more readily laughs at herself, and seeks out and enjoys the company of peers more? Yes! And because of that, our family is just, well, happier too.

Don't get me wrong, we still have our days and moments. Lilly, without a doubt, is on the spectrum; her mind clearly works differently; she clearly has social impairments and anxieties. She will never be "cured" and we know that. We have good *days (many) and bad days (few). However, thanks to these interventions, we are able to focus more on our daughter and less on her impairments.*

What is it that we want for our daughter now? Well, it's no different than what any parent wants for their "typical" child, really. We want her to be happy, we want her to be fulfilled and lead a purposeful life, we want her to have meaningful relationships, and we want her to be understood and appreciated. We credit these interventions with allowing us to be on the typical journey of parenthood, just like everyone else.

—Cindy and Doug, parents of Lilly

● ● ● ● ● ● ● ● ● ●

SUMMARY

A largely or totally Incidental Intervention strategy works best for children 2.5–3 years and older scoring 2.5 or higher on the Autism Intervention Responsiveness Scale (see Chapter 4, Figure 4.1). Such youngsters usually exhibit higher intellectual ability and stronger verbal skills and may be hyperlexic. They often exhibit considerable social interest but display limited social skills. They tend to have few hyperactivity and inattentiveness concerns, and some, but not extreme, anxiety. They generally engage in very little or no repetitive, stereotyped behavior but may have extreme compulsive routines and perfectionism. Lilly is a typical example, whose main challenges revolved around her lack of empathy and social perceptiveness combined with an intense need for control and perfectionism. In working with such capable children, it is useful to bear in mind Mark Twain's dictum: "Habit is habit and not to be flung out of the window by any man, but coaxed downstairs a step at a time." (1894/2006).

REFERENCES

Attwood, T. (2004). *Exploring feelings: Anxiety: Cognitive Behaviour Therapy to manage anxiety.* Arlington, TX: Future Horizons.

Gilliam, J.E. (2006). *Gilliam Autism Rating Scale–Second Edition (GARS-2).* Austin, TX:PRO-ED.

Halle, J.W., Baer, D.M., & Spradlin, J.E. (1981). Teachers' generalized use of delay as a stimulus control procedure to increase language use in handicapped children. *Journal of Applied Behavior Analysis, 14*(4), 389.

Hart, B., & Risley, T.R. (1968). Establishing the use of descriptive adjectives in the spontaneous speech of disadvantaged children. *Journal of Applied Behavior Analysis, 1,* 109–120.

Hart, B., & Risley, T.R. (1975). Incidental teaching of language in the preschool. *Journal of Applied Behavior Analysis, 8*(4), 411–420.

Kaiser, A.P. (1993). Parent-implemented language intervention: An environmental perspective. In A.P. Kaiser & D.B. Gray (Eds.), *Enhancing children's communication: Research foundations of intervention* (pp. 63–84). Baltimore: Paul H. Brookes Publishing Co.

Koegel, R.L., Bimbela, A., & Schreibman, L. (1996). Collateral effects of parent training on family interactions. *Journal of Autism and Developmental Disorders, 26*(3), 347–359.

Koegel, R.I., & Frea, W.D. (1993). Treatment of social behavior in autism through the modification of pivotal social skills. *Journal of Applied Behavior Analysis, 26*(3), 369–377.

Koegel, R.L., & Koegel, L.K. (2006). *Pivotal response treatments for autism: Communication, social, and academic development.* Baltimore: Paul H. Brookes Publishing Co.

Lord, C., Rutter, M., DiLavore, P.C., & Risi, S. (1999). *Autism Diagnostic Observation Schedule–WPS Edition.* Los Angeles: Western Psychological Services.

McGee, G.G., Almeida, M.C., Sulzer-Azaroff, B., & Feldman, R.S. (1992). Promoting reciprocal interactions via peer incidental teaching. *Journal of Applied Behavior Analysis, 25,* 117–126.

McGee, G.G., Krantz, P.J., & McClannahan, L.E. (1985). The facilitative effects of incidental teaching on preposition use by autistic children. *Journal of Applied Behavior Analysis, 18*(1), 17.

McWilliam, R.A., & Scott, S. (2001). A support approach to early intervention: A three-part framework. *Infants & Young Children, 13*(4), 55.

Noonan, M.J., & McCormick, L. (1993). *Early intervention in natural environments: Methods and procedures.* Florence, KY: Brooks/Cole.

Partington, J.W. (2007). *Assessment of basic language and learning skills-revised (ABLLS-R).* Walnut Creek, CA: The Behavior Analysts.

Peterson, P. (2004). Naturalistic language teaching procedures for children at risk for delays. *The Behavior Analyst Today, 5*(4), 404–424.

Pierce, K., & Schreibman, L. (1995). Increasing complex social behaviors in children with autism: Effects of peer-implemented pivotal response training. *Journal of Applied Behavior Analysis, 28,* 285–295.

Rogers-Warren, A., & Warren, S.F. (1980). Mands for verbalization: Facilitating the display of newly trained language in children. *Behavior Modification, 4*(3), 361.

Schopler, E., Van Bourgondien, M.E., Wellman, G.J., & Love, S.R. (2010). *Childhood Autism Rating Scale* (2nd ed.). Los Angeles: Western Psychological Services.

Sundberg, M.L. (2008). *Verbal behavior milestones assessment and placement program (VB-MAPP).* Concord, CA: Advancements in Verbal Behavior Press.

Twain, M. (2006). *The tragedy of Puddn'head Wilson* [Electronic version]. Retrieved March 31, 2010, from http://www.gutenberg.org/files/102/102-h/102-h.htm#2HCH0006 (Original work published 1894)

Warren, S.F., & Gazdag, G. (1990). Facilitating early language development with milieu intervention procedures. *Journal of Early Intervention, 14,* 62–86.

Warren, S.F., & Kaiser, A.P. (1986). Incidental language teaching: A critical review. *Journal of Speech and Hearing Disorders, 51,* 291–299.

Warren, S.F., McQuarter, R.J., & Rogers-Warren, A.P. (1984). The effects of mands and models on the speech of unresponsive language-delayed preschool children. *Journal of Speech and Hearing Disorders, 49,* 43–52.

Wilde, O. (2009). Act I, Scene 1. *An ideal husband* [Electronic version]. Retrieved April 10, 2010, from http://www.gutenberg.org/files/885/885-h/885-h.htm (Original work published 1912)

9

Blended Interventions for Younger Children with Uneven Skills and Marked Restricted Repetitive Behavior

with Beth Burggraff and Lisa M. Barsness

> *""The qualities or modes of things do never really exist each of them apart by itself, and separated from all others, but are mixed, as it were, and blended together, several in the same object."*

—George Berkeley, *A Treatise Concerning Principles of Human Knowledge* (1710/2009)

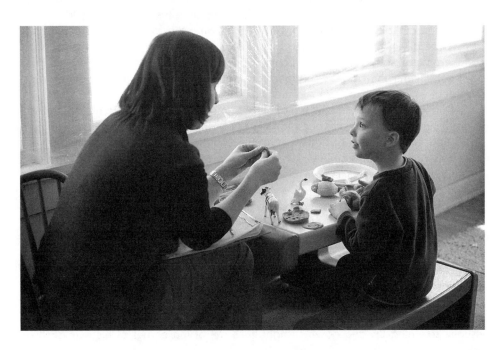

● ● ● ● ● ● ● ● ● ●

INTRODUCTION: LEO

Leo was 4 years old when we first met him and his parents during a visit to our clinic. He had a captivating smile, medium brown hair, and alert blue eyes. Leo had been receiving Relationship Development Intervention four times per week as well as occupational therapy services and early childhood special education services. His mother's eyes teared as she described Leo "frantically running around his pre-school classroom like a frightened, caged bird" as though he were unable to escape from a terrifying situation. His parents were seeking a calmer, more structured one-to-one intervention that would promote Leo's skills and reduce his emotional upsets and behavioral challenges.

His parents said Leo was excessively active and difficult to discipline. Leo found it difficult to focus, flitting frequently from one toy or activity to another after only seconds had elapsed. Activity transitions were difficult, and Leo had food intolerances and sleep difficulties as well. His compulsive rituals were striking, such as insisting that he carry around a toy dog named "Goya" and a toy cat named "Laura," literally at all times. If he needed to use one hand for another activity, he shoved one of the toy animals under his arm, pressed against his body, until his hand was free again to hold the animal. If an adult attempted to extricate one of the animals so he could participate in another activity, he cried, hit, and tried to run away. If one of the animals were inadvertently mislaid, a frenzied housewide search would ensue until the object of his compulsive ritual was found.

Leo's mother, Deanna, is a professional photographer. His father, David, is an accomplished visual artist. Both parents are spontaneous, creative people who are integrative thinkers. When Leo was upset and crying, that was especially difficult for his parents to tolerate.

During multidisciplinary testing at another clinic, Leo obtained cognitive, socio-emotional, and adaptive behavior scores of borderline impaired, and a language score of low average. His score on an autism screening test was in the mild to moderate range of the autism spectrum. Leo's scores on a test for possible mental health signs were all in the normal range based on teacher report, but parents reported that there were significant physical complaints and attention problems. The psychologist conducting the assessment concluded that Leo's history and symptoms were consistent with a diagnosis of Autistic Disorder.

During our initial clinic observation and interview, Leo clung to his mother and had difficulty separating. He occasionally established fleeting eye contact with therapists near him on the floor of the playroom. Leo didn't initiate interactions with our therapists or with the examiner. His mother reported that he had interest in peers but didn't know how to initiate or maintain social play. He fussed and whined throughout much of the session. Our senior behavior therapist, who would subsequently be working with Leo, had difficulty engaging him in activities, though he showed some interest in one or two toys. His mother reported that he reacted inappropriately to others' emotions. For example, he laughed when his little brother, Henry, was crying.

Leo showed no reaction to questions directed to him by adults during our observation. His mother reported that he often repeated phrases from books and videos out of context. She also said Leo seldom took part in imaginative play. Leo displayed several unique stereotypic behaviors, such as lining up objects, or *edging*—visually scanning up and down straight lines out of the corner of his eye, such as the verge of the ceiling and wall or the edge of a rug on the floor of the assessment room. When parents or therapists attempted to divert his attention away from a preferred activity to a new pursuit, he cried, screamed, and shoved or hit.

On the AIRS™ (Figure 9.1; see Chapter 4, Figure 4.1), Leo scored 1.7, suggesting he would likely profit from a Blended Intervention (from 1.5 to 2.49), beginning with DTI and gradually shifting to Incidental Intervention strategies. Leo's AIRS profile indicates special challenges in Joint Attention, Insistence on Sameness, and Activity Level, which will likely require a more structured DTI approach. Most of his other scale scores are consistent with beginning with a DTI approach and transitioning slowly to an incidental intervention strategy.

THERAPY PRINCIPLES AND ASSUMPTIONS

Children with uneven skill profiles like Leo with greater challenges in several domains often profit from an initial DTI approach and gradual transitioning to Incidental Intervention as skills are consolidated. Initially, greater structure and predictability clarify expectations to the child and reduce anxiety. ABA Discrete Trial principles and techniques are the foundation upon which incidental strategies are subsequently layered.

Roots in Applied Behavior Analysis and Incidental Teaching

Blended Intervention for younger children with limited social skills and borderline-to-average language and cognitive skills, and who display marked restricted repetitive behavior like Leo, involves a combination of DTI and Incidental Intervention strategies. Because Leo had an extremely short attention span, followed almost no adult verbal directions, and had extensive compulsive behavior and restricted interests, we decided to begin his therapy using DTI.

Following 2 weeks of rapport building, Leo's therapists began introducing short DTI intervals (e.g., 5 to 10 minutes) using established principles and procedures (Leaf, McEachin, & Harsh, 1999; Maurice, Green, & Luce, 1996). These were interpolated with short free-play periods with access to one of his favorite toys. Clear verbal and gestural cues were presented by the therapist, beginning with "Leo, come sit," accompanied by pointing to the chair while touching the chair with a finger. In the beginning, preferred edible treats (e.g., raisins or other fruit, cereal) were used, alternating with praise and "high fives" as reinforcers. Leo initially failed to follow adult directions, so he was gently guided to the chair while the instruction, "Leo, come sit," was given, accompanied

2.5–3.0												
2.0–2.49												
1.5–1.99												
1.0–1.49												
Domain	COM	JAT	IMT	SNT	INS	NIT	RMB	INT	ATT	ACT	ANX	PHS

Figure 9.1. Leo's baseline Autism Intervention Responsiveness Scale (AIRS™) Profile. (*Key:* COM, Communication; JAT, Joint Attention; IMT, Imitation; SNT, Social Interest; INS, Insistence on Sameness; NIT, Narrow Interests; RMB, Repetitive Motor Behavior; INT, Intellectual Ability; ATT, Attention; ACT, Activity; ANX, Anxiety/Fearfulnes; PHS, Physical Features)

by pointing with the other hand. Once he had begun to sit when requested, he was taught to imitate hand and arm movements, such as "clap hands, rub tummy, and pat head," using small edible treats as reinforcers. He was also taught to make appropriate movements with several toys, such as driving a car across the table and rocking the baby. The therapist said, "Leo, do this" and clapped her hands or rocked the doll baby. As soon as he made an imitative approximation, the therapist said, "Great job, Leo; you clapped your hands," and offered him an animal cracker. Functional actions that fit into daily routines, such as grasping a spoon and bringing it to his mouth, were first introduced as DTI goals and then implemented incidentally by his parents.

Embedding Trials within Play Themes and Daily Activities

Leo was next taught to follow simple directions, such as "Put it there," "Give it to me," "Put it away" (e.g., a toy), or "Hang it up" (e.g., an article of clothing). These were selected because his parents were eager for him to learn to follow directions that would be helpful in his daily family life and in preschool. He spontaneously began making verbal requests, such as "More juice!" or "More tickles!" Therapy staff initially reinforced any request immediately, then introduced a delay and visually prompted him to establish eye contact by moving their finger from in front of his eyes to their own eyes in one continuous movement. Over days and weeks, he gradually increased eye contact when making verbal requests, and prompts were no longer necessary.

Leo had several preferred play activities, one of which was structured around a complex farm set that included a barn, silo, chicken house, male and female farmers, various types of animals (cows, calf, horses, pony, pigs, sheep, goats, chickens, dog, cat), tractors, other farm implements, fencing, and trees. Imaginative farm thematic activities were often initiated by Leo but subsequently were semistructured by therapists. A therapist suggested a specific activity, such as feeding the cows or plowing the field. These scenario-based activities were used to teach receptive and expressive labeling of prepositions (*in, on, under, on top, below, beside, inside*): Therapist: "Where is the cow?" Leo: "In the barn." Therapist: "Put the pig in the pen." Leo puts the pig within the fenced area (McGee, Krantz, & McClannahan, 1985).

The farm scenario was also used to teach relational and category concepts, such as *big or small* and *animals versus machines:* Therapist: "Where is the big horse?" Leo points to the larger horse. Therapist: "Let's put all the animals here and the machines there," (accompanied by pointing). Leo begins to sort the toys into animals and machine categories.

Leo was taught to name and make actions, first by a therapist demonstrating and labeling the actions—such as clapping, throwing, or waving—and then having Leo name the action when it was demonstrated (*stimulus*: therapist clapping hands; *response*: Leo says, "Clapping"; *reinforcer*: therapist says, "Right, I was clapping," gives Leo a tickle, and offers him a pretzel). Next, Leo was shown photos on cards of similar actions, but also including other actions such as running, sitting, shouting, batting, pouring, and so on, and was reinforced for correctly labeling them. When Leo was proficient in labeling pictures on cards, his parents were encouraged to read picture books to Leo and ask him to identify actions of characters in the books, such as *Green Eggs and Ham* (Seuss, 1960; e.g., Dad: "What is Sam I Am doing?" Child: "Riding in car!" Dad: "Right, he's riding in a car."). Over time, most of the reinforcers were social or access to preferred activities (see Hart & Risley, 1982).

Leo often had difficulty dealing with transitions, so therapy staff introduced a *picture schedule* to reduce ambiguity and allow him to anticipate events that were coming next. Initially there were two pictures on the schedule; one activity such as imitating toy play was followed by the second, a reinforcing activity such as playing a chase game with the therapist. After he was comfortable and performing reliably with a two-step picture schedule, third and fourth pictures were added, in each case making certain he was successfully following the schedule before adding more activities. The order of the pictures was changed regularly so Leo wouldn't adopt a rigid routine. Later, the therapist asked Leo what pictures *he* would like to place on the schedule. There were five Velcro tabs attached to a vertical cardboard column onto which he could place pictures from a pool of 10 activity photos. When it was necessary to include a specific activity, the therapist placed that photo on the schedule first and Leo added the rest. Once Leo had become accustomed to the picture schedule during therapy, his parents constructed similar schedules around other daily routines, such as getting ready for bed, bathing, and preparing for school.

Learning Is Initially Incremental and Rapid Later

Leo experienced limited progress on his individualized treatment plan goals for the first few months. After reviewing his low rate of learning new skills and studying the details of our intervention method, we decided to make a transition from intervention exclusively within the DTI format at a child-sized table to beginning to embed the same type of activities within familiar routines or situations—a Blended Intervention. Almost immediately, Leo's progress sharply increased. Subsequently, Leo's intervention was largely conducted within typical daily routines or thematic imaginative play activities. Only when first introducing a new activity was a DTI approach used.

Among the goals added were playing board games (e.g., The Very Hungry Caterpillar) and fine- and gross-motor games (e.g., Don't Spill the Beans and Tag), which involved alternating turns, first with his therapists, then his parents, and later with same-age peers. We then added social goals involving recognition of emotions from facial expressions and describing events in a scene or activity and recalling them later. Circumstances that led to different emotions were taught next, like receiving a present leading to happiness and a child's cat running away leading to sadness. Next Leo learned concrete and more abstract classes based on form, features, and functions. For example, he learned the classes of animals with four versus those with two legs, things that fly versus things that do not fly, or food versus non-food items.

Capitalizing on the Child's Interests and Aptitudes

Leo has surprisingly good language skills compared with many children on the autism spectrum. Sometimes he could be a real chatterbox. For example, while playing with Play-Doh, Leo said, "It's a river. Make a bridge over the river. The water is going under the bridge. Now you make a tree. Birds can sit in the tree."

Structure Learning Opportunities

Though most of Leo's intervention had been switched from discrete trials to learning embedded within ongoing, naturally occurring events, to ensure adequate therapy intensity some discrete trials were inserted into typical daily routines that he found especially interesting. Leo had become progressively interested in playing with other children, so he was taught specific skills in initiating a social interaction, which included first observing what the other children were doing and then commenting to the peers about their activity before attempting to join in (see McGee & Daly, 2007). "What are they playing?" the therapist asked Leo. "Playing cars," he replied. "That's right, Leo," the therapist replied. "Say something nice about their cars, Leo." "Cars go fast!" Leo chimed in. He practiced saying several types of leading comments to help initiate an interaction. A therapist accompanied him to preschool and, for several weeks, prompted him in initiating conversations and then entering into peers' play. After he was doing so successfully, the therapists gradually faded their prompts and let nature take its course, as his peers reinforced his attempts to play with them by saying, "Want to play cars, Leo?"

Overcoming Compulsive Routines

Leo had numerous compulsive rituals, notably, insisting on holding Goya and Laura, his toy dog and cat. After about 6 months, therapists asked Leo to place Goya on the table "so he could watch while we play." The therapist explained, "Goya can't see what we are doing when you are holding him." Eventually, Goya was put in a toy bed so he could take a nap while Leo worked with his therapist. The same procedure was used with the toy cat. Several months of using this *fading* procedure were required to gradually remove the two toy animals completely from therapy. When Leo was especially anxious about leaving preferred toys during therapy, he learned to say to himself, "Time for school. You can play with the animals after school. They need to rest. It's school time now." Leo's parents adopted the same procedure when therapists were not present. Periodically, Leo remembered one of his animals and said, "Goya is resting." Leo continues to have other compulsive rituals, which are being approached similarly.

Capitalizing on Social Interest

From the outset, it was obvious Leo was very socially interested. He soon looked forward to his therapists arriving at his home, and when peer play dates began he seemed excited and at times elated. Peers were prompted to help Leo by being "helpers" and were given instructions quietly so Leo was unable to hear the instruction (sometimes whispered in their ear). At the beginning of a peer play session, the peer was reminded of goals for the session ("Try to wait until Leo looks at you before you answer a question"). Gestures were also used (pointing to Leo if the peer asks the therapist a question about a toy or item, or the therapist may use an "I don't know" gesture to prompt the peer to direct comments to Leo). When making a schedule of activities for peer play sessions, both Leo and the peer were able to make choices for activities to keep interest level high for both children. At the end of the peer play session, the peer was encouraged to pick from a treasure box of items.

Data Intensity

Because Leo's intervention initially involved largely DTI methods, the same intensity of data collection was used as in Chapter 7, particularly early in therapy. As therapy made the transition to more Incidental Intervention, probe measures were periodically taken, because there are no predictable trials as the basis for data collection. Some data collected during Incidental Intervention is entirely spontaneous and often depends on others' behavior, such as peers in day care. Therapists carried a clipboard and a prepared data sheet with them at all times during therapy to record such spontaneous events. At times, therapists contrived opportunities, such as making gestures and recording whether Leo responded appropriately to their gestures (such as shrugging shoulders and extending palms up, meaning "I don't know" or "I'm confused"). Therapists wore two tally counters on their belts, one to tally each request and the other to tally requests with eye contact. This made it possible to evaluate the total number of verbal requests Leo made, and the proportion in which Leo used appropriate eye contact.

Setting: Home, School, and Community

For the first 6 months of therapy, intervention was largely indoors at home and in the family's backyard. His parents enrolled Leo in day care and preschool programs to provide opportunities for Leo to learn to interact with peers. Our therapists attended day care with Leo for the first few months to ensure that he learned necessary skills to interact with his peers, such as responding when spoken to, taking turns, and sharing. Over time therapists participated progressively less as Leo became more proficient in his communication and social skills.

Assessment

As in previous chapters, criterion referenced skills assessments were done to determine baseline skills and monitor ongoing progress. Figure 9.2 shows Leo's performance on the first nine scales of the ABLLS-R (Partington, 2007) at baseline (dark) and after 1 year of intervention (light). Note that in some domains, Leo began with strong skills, such as Receptive Language, Vocal Imitation, and Spontaneous Vocalizations. On others, such as Visual Performance, Motor Imitation, and Making Requests, his entry skills were very limited, so these became focal areas for his individualized treatment plan (detailed in the next section). Over the first year of intervention, he made substantial gains in Visual Performance, Motor Imitation, and Labeling, as indicated by the bars in light gray.

● ● ● ● ● ● ● ● ● ●

LEO: A CHILD WHO THRIVED ON BLENDED DISCRETE TRIAL AND INCIDENTAL INTERVENTION

As noted earlier, Leo's therapy was initially largely DTI but soon made the transition to a combination of DTI and Incidental Intervention.

Individualized Treatment Plan

Leo's AIRS™ score of 1.7 placed him in the lower end of the Blended Intervention range. Children scoring 1.5 to 1.9 may require DTI intervention to begin therapy for the first few months and may continue to require a DTI strategy whenever a new goal is introduced. Once they have learned basic skills, they can often make the transition to largely Incidental Intervention. Prizant and Wetherby (1998) aptly suggested such a strategy is suitable for some children.

In part, based on the results of the baseline ABLLS-R assessment (Partington, 2007) together with observations during initial rapport building and discussions with parents regarding their priorities, a set of initial intervention goals and objectives was established focusing on the three primary diagnostic domains that characterize differences among children with ASDs: socialization, communication, and restricted repetitive behavior. Leo's individualized treatment plan goals (Figure 9.3)

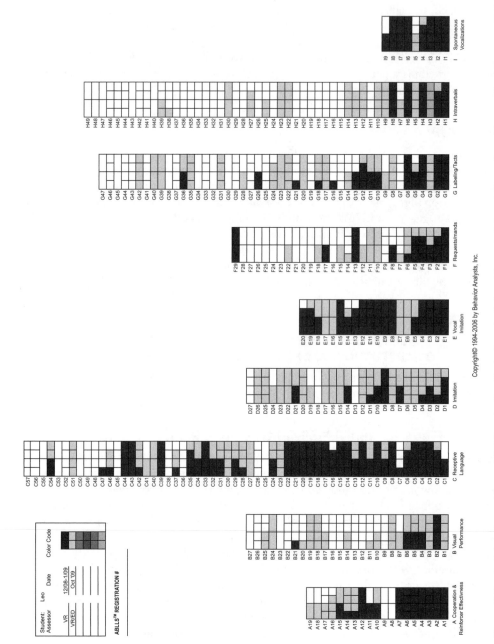

Figure 9.2. Leo's baseline and 1-year ABLLS-R results. Baseline is shown in dark and 1 year in light, revealing substantial gains. (From Partington, J.W. [2007]. *Assessment of Basic Language and Learning Skills-Revised [ABLLS-R].* Walnut Creek, CA: The Behavior Analysts, Inc.; adapted by permission.)

Treatment Goals and Objectives

Child's name: _Leo_____   Date of birth: _____

Parent(s) name(s): _Deanna_____   Date: _9/1/09_____

I. Socialization

Long-term goal	**Appropriate gross motor game play**
Short-term goal	When playing a gross motor game, Leo will play appropriately with 1 adult prompt or less, 80% of the time, across 3 consecutive sessions for at least 10 games.
Strategies/treatment methods	Practitioners/parents will use a variety of prompting techniques including modeling, visual supports, and contextual cues to teach appropriate gross motor game play. Prompts will be faded and differential reinforcement will be used for independent responses. Use social reinforcement specific to the game.

Date introduced	9/1/09	Projected mastery date	5/1/10

Long-term goal	**Imitates peers**
Short-term goal	When playing with peers, Leo will follow instructions from adult or through playing games to imitate peers (e.g., Simon Says, Follow the Leader) appropriately with 1 adult prompt or less, 80% of the time across 3 consecutive sessions for at least 3 different peers.
Strategies/treatment methods	Practitioners/parents will use a variety of prompting techniques including modeling, visual supports, and contextual cues to teach imitation of peers. Prompts will be faded and differential reinforcement will be used for independent responses. Initially use verbal praise, but fade to the natural reinforcer of the peer's reaction to imitation.

Date introduced	2/3/10	Projected mastery date	5/1/10

Long-term goal	**Responds to "stop" request from peers**
Short-term goal	When asked to "stop" by a peer, Leo will discontinue behavior without adult prompts 80% of the time across 3 consecutive sessions.

Figure 9.3. Leo's individualized Treatment Goals and Objectives plan.

(continued)

Treatment Goals and Objectives *(continued)*

Strategies/treatment methods	Across all functional teaching environments, practitioners/parents will use a variety of prompting strategies to teach responding to stop. Prompts will be faded as independence with skill increases. Use praise such as "good job, you stopped!" then fade praise.		
Date introduced	2/3/10	Projected mastery date	5/1/10

Long-term goal	**Reciprocal statements**		
Short-term goal	When a parent, practitioner, or peer makes a comment (statement), Leo will respond with a contingent comment 80% of the time across 3 consecutive assessments for at least 5 different topic statements.		
Strategies/treatment methods	Practitioners will use a variety of prompting techniques to assist Leo in identifying conversational topic (e.g., 3-D objects, photos, books) and responding reciprocally (visual, verbal, gestural cues). Prompts will be faded and differential reinforcement will be provided for responding. Partner's contingent comment will serve as reinforcing consequence.		
Date introduced	2/3/10	Projected mastery date	5/1/10

II. Communication

Long-term goal	**Uses pronouns correctly**		
Short-term goal	Leo will label 8 pronouns, both receptively and expressively, in 80% of opportunities independently across 3 consecutive assessments.		
Strategies/treatment methods	In all teaching environments, practitioners/parents will prompt Leo to use appropriate pronouns, gradually fading prompts and utilizing differential reinforcement for all unprompted responses. Use affirmation and praise as reinforcers.		
Date introduced	10/31/09	Projected mastery date	5/1/10

Long-term goal	**Recalls events**		
Short-term goal	When asked, "What did you do" or "Who did you see?" Leo will be able to describe a previous event or person 80% of the time across 3 consecutive assessments.		

Strategies/treatment methods	Across all functional teaching environments, practitioners/parents will use a variety of prompting strategies to teach the recalling events. Visual supports may be used initially. Prompts will be faded as independence with recalling events increases. Reinforcement will consist of telling Leo what he said was interesting, or saying "Wow, that was great!" and so forth.		
Date introduced	1/28/10	Projected mastery date	5/1/10

Long-term goal	**Identifies what's wrong** (Corresponds to discharge objectives 11-18)		
Short-term goal	When presented with a picture that is obviously incorrect or an emergency and asked, "What's wrong?" Leo will identify the problem correctly 80% of the time across 3 consecutive assessments.		
Strategies/treatment methods	In all teaching environments, practitioners/parents will prompt Leo to correctly label incorrect items or emergency situations, gradually fading prompts and utilizing differential reinforcement for all unprompted responses. Reinforcement will be social, verbal praise for identifying what was wrong.		
Date introduced	2/3/10	Projected mastery date	5/1/10

III. Restricted, Repetitive, and Stereotyped Behavior

Long-term goal	**Follows schedule to get ready**		
Short-term goal	Leo will follow a schedule to get ready for a community outing, with one adult prompt or less, for up to 5 written items, 80% of the opportunities across 3 consecutive assessments.		
Strategies/treatment methods	Practitioners will target this skill in a 1:1 therapy setting before implementing in the natural environment. Practitioners will gradually fade prompts and use differential reinforcement for independent responses. Leo will initially be reinforced following each step in the schedule, then every other step, and finally all steps. Tangible reinforcers will be faded to social reinforcement.		
Date introduced	9/1/09	Projected mastery date	5/1/10

Long-term goal	**Tolerance of denial** (Corresponds with discharge objectives 19–22)		

(continued)

Treatment Goals and Objectives *(continued)*

Short-term goal	When requesting an item, Leo will tolerate denial of item without engaging in aggression toward others or verbally protesting longer than 5 seconds 80% of the time across 3 consecutive assessment opportunities.
Strategies/treatment methods	Practitioners will target this skill in a 1:1 therapy setting initially, using reinforcement pairing techniques as well as redirection to preferred tasks. Use gradually increasing delay combined with larger tangible reinforcer for tolerating longer delays, and brief social reinforcement for tolerating only short delays.

Date introduced	2/3/10	Projected mastery date	5/1/10

IV. Family Skills Goals

Long-term goal	**Parents will teach age-appropriate daily living skills**
Short-term goal	Leo's parents will teach 4 age-appropriate daily living skills (e.g., dressing and bathing), with minimal assistance from the senior behavior therapist or treatment supervisor, over a 6-month period.

addressed more advanced skills in all three autism domains. Behavior therapists and Leo's parents, under the guidance of senior behavior therapists and the supervising psychologist, implemented all activities.

Sample Outcomes

For the first 6 months, Leo's parents had been concerned that 30 hours of therapy per week would be too difficult for him to tolerate and requested that it be limited to 15 hours per week. Although Leo was making progress, it was considerably slower than we had thought was appropriate to make the gains necessary to prepare him for a successful school transition (see Cowan & Allen, 2007). Leo's parents came to realize he greatly enjoyed working with our therapists, and rather than finding it stressful, he spent much of his therapy time laughing and having fun. At that point they requested therapy intensity be increased to 30 to 35 hours per week. After that, Leo's skill acquisition really took off. The graphs in Figures 9.4–9.7 illustrate outcomes after 1 year in four skill areas.

Following Picture Schedule

A picture schedule was used to facilitate transitions between activities and reduce Leo's resistance to change. Leo's baseline of following pictures placed on a schedule board before being taught to use the picture schedule was zero (i.e., he was unable to use the picture schedule). Leo's performance on a three-picture schedule is shown in Figure 9.4 in the three points on the far left. The middle portion of the

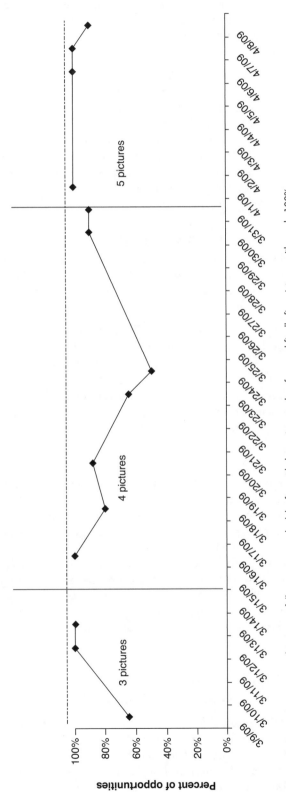

Figure 9.4. Leo's progress in learning to follow a picture schedule, first with three pictures, then four, and finally five pictures, with nearly 100% accuracy.

graph shows Leo's performance on a four-picture schedule, and the final four points on the right show Leo's performance on a five-picture schedule. Once he mastered the picture schedule during therapy, his parents also used picture schedules to support transitions around typical daily routines.

Turn-Taking

Turn-taking is a pivotal social skill that promotes interactions with peers (Koegel & Frea, 1993). Leo was taught to take turns, initially with therapists, then parents, and finally peers. Initially Leo seemed to think it was always his turn when playing games. By first providing Leo with three or four turns in a row at a game, then having the therapist take one turn, however, Leo gradually was taught to tolerate others having their turn. Eventually the ratio would be two or three Leo turns and one therapist turn and, finally, turns alternated. His progress is shown in Figure 9.5.

Labels Action Shown in Pictures

Leo was first taught to label an action made by one of the therapists, such as throwing, jumping, or running. Then he was taught to label actions in videos. When he was successful, he was finally taught to label actions in still pictures (Figure 9.6).

Identifies Categories

Over 6 months, Leo learned 18 categories of objects to a criterion of at least 80% correct over multiple occasions with multiple therapists and his parents. Figure 9.7 shows Leo's progress in learning to label categories of objects, such as animals, vehicles, and plants. Initially categories that were very dissimilar were taught, such as people versus vehicles. Eventually, categories with more similarities were introduced, such as zoo animals versus farm animals.

Generalization of Skills to the Family

Therapists facilitated generalization from staff to parents by first demonstrating to Mom and Dad how the skill had been taught and how to evaluate whether Leo's response was appropriate. Then parents were encouraged to try the same activity on their own and report back on how it went. The dialogue with the parents about the new skill was continued until Leo was independent with that skill with the two of them. Adjustments were made along the way as necessary. Changes in how therapists were teaching new skills were discussed at the team meeting in which both parents participated, which further promoted transfer of skills from therapy staff to parents. An example is teaching Leo to follow a written schedule. Mom and Dad were able to use this, with their own modifications, with great success at home and in the community.

Family's Perspective: Leo

I shudder when I think about the first year and a half after Leo was diagnosed with autism. It was such a confusing and lonely time. Leo was soon to be 3 years old, and although we tried to do everything possible for early intervention, it was obvious it still wasn't enough. My husband and I felt like the only people on the planet who understood and enjoyed Leo for the bright little boy he was. I was afraid no

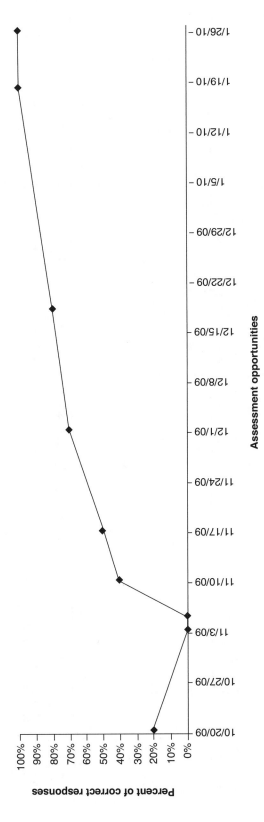

Figure 9.5. Leo's progress in learning the social skill of taking turns. After a small reversal early in teaching this goal, he acquired the skill to 100% tolerance for alternating turns.

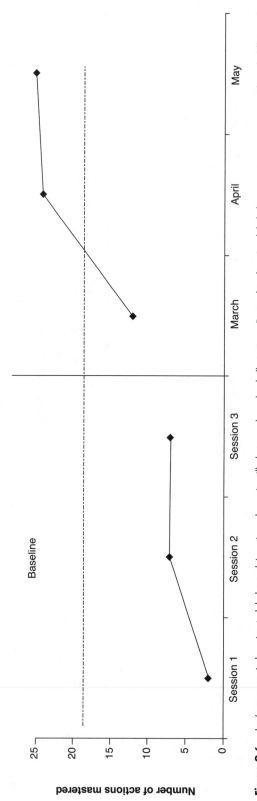

Figure 9.6. Leo's progress in learning to label people's actions shown in still photographs or book illustrations. During baseline, Leo labeled as many as seven actions. Through differential reinforcement of labeling a wider array of actions, he was able to label 25 different actions.

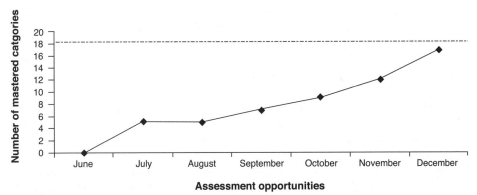

Figure 9.7.   Leo learned to identify 18 categories of things over 6 months, after establishing a zero baseline of this skill. Recognition of categories is an important part of semantic knowledge used in conversation.

one besides us would ever know him, because at the time he didn't allow anyone else in his world.

Although Leo does have trouble with functional language, he was an early talker and detailed, descriptive language has always been one of his strengths. At 2 years old he was speaking in sentences. He knew the alphabet, colors, and shapes before he was 2. He devoured books, was very observant, and has always loved to learn. He was happy, playful, and loved imaginary play. All these wonderful qualities he could easily express within the walls of our home, with only his mom and dad.

The trouble was having a life outside of our home and helping Leo tolerate unpreferred activities. Leo would become very obsessive, agitated, and nervous in public places. He was a wreck at holiday gatherings and would hide in any empty room he could find. Going on simple outings like the park became a nightmare. Time at the park was spent chasing him, as he would bolt in any direction he could find, running away from the park. Our dear nanny at the time, having run out of ideas to entertain him, would just drive around all day with Leo in her car. He was happy as can be, strapped securely in his seat, in a controlled environment, talking about all the wonderful things he saw. I remember the enormous gas tabs we reimbursed her for.

We knew there must be a better way to help Leo, but we had no idea of our other options. For a year, Leo was already receiving autism early intervention services with the public school district. The services available for Leo amounted to 2 hours of occupational therapy a month, 2 hours of speech therapy a month, and 3 hours of autism intervention a week.

One of my saddest memories of that hard time was watching Leo just run and run and run around the room of his autism early intervention preschool. He looked miserable and overwhelmed, like a trapped bird trying to find a way out. There were fluorescent lights buzzing and groups of people having different conversations. Circle time consisted of a song playing on the boom box; the teachers and students were supposed to sing along while using felt boards to describe the song. As an adult without autism, I was overwhelmed with all the commotion in the room; I could only imagine what it felt like for Leo.

I've always received the best information about resources from other parents of children with autism. I was sharing my concerns with another mother and she highly recommended MEAP [Minnesota Early Autism Project]. I researched MEAP and spoke with other parents who were thrilled to have their child work with them. All I knew is that everything I heard about, I wanted for Leo. I just knew in my heart it was the right place for Leo, and I wasn't wrong. I think I called them every day for 3 months until they finally had an opening. They were probably so tired of my calls.

MEAP's staff has always treated Leo as a smart kid who happens to have autism. He is not just a diagnosis with qualities to fix, but he is seen as an individual who is enjoyed, respected, and understood by the therapists he works with. Through play and learning about Leo's preferred activities, they spent the first couple months becoming the coolest people in the world to Leo, and they succeeded. Creating this foundation of fun and play was very motivating for him. Within the first 2 weeks, he was putty in their hands. The difference in therapy was astonishing. From our perspective, it was the first time we witnessed effective therapy for Leo, and he was responding so well. We noticed how motivated he was to work with his therapists, and he really wanted their approval. Leo was tolerating activities that he refused to do with anyone else in the past. He was becoming more focused and maintained interest in activities for longer periods of time.

I really appreciate how the therapists move around during their sessions. They take Leo to the park, in our yard, all over the house. He is never bored and they always keep it interesting for him. Leo works with up to five different therapists, and this helps him learn to be flexible with different personalities, styles, and ways of playing certain games. It's more likely to help him transition to a school setting at a later date.

Leo looked forward to his sessions with excitement and responded really well to the dramatic increase of hours, which went from 4 hours a week to 35 hours with MEAP. The more time with them the better, seemed to be his attitude.

Leo used to recoil from past therapists. They were basically strangers to him, who came to our house periodically, touched him, asked him to do certain things for an hour, then packed up and left. The preschool was too stressful for him and he needed to start social groups at a slower pace. The past therapists with public special ed. were well-trained and very kind. However, the resources offered could only take their therapy so far. We found that Leo thrived when he could build a relationship with his therapists in a one-on-one setting.

MEAP is wonderful at bringing Leo into the community. Their approach is to keep him successful, so they work with what he can handle socially and build up from there. Currently, Leo's therapists shadow him at a preschool and two play groups and facilitate play dates. All the sessions are with typically developing children. Leo is not anywhere as anxious as he used to be. He really enjoys the play groups, and having a trusted therapist with him helps him navigate and understand social situations.

I'm also happy to report that we don't think twice about going to the park now. We all have fun and he enjoys the playground and other children. We had a dinner party at our house recently and he sang for our guests and was quite the entertainer. We actually went to holiday parties this year. Leo brought a puzzle to keep him occupied and when another child took his piece, he smiled at the child and told him that they could share. We're really proud of him. We're also happy to be gaining some of our social life back as well.

We have been working with MEAP for well over a year now and already our life has changed for the better. They not only help Leo but also support our family to be more successful in raising Leo. We feel we can talk to them openly, and if difficult *behaviors come up, they help us navigate and find solutions. Life is not as lonely or confusing as it once was. Everyone involved is committed to helping Leo succeed. With team meetings twice a month and quarterly meetings with the staff psychologist while we're with MEAP, there are no longer any cracks or craters for Leo to fall through. We now have a tightly woven net to help Leo gain footing for the rest of his life. We still have a long way to go, but Leo is happy and that makes his mom and dad even happier.*

—Deanna, mother of Leo

● ● ● ● ● ● ● ● ● ●

SUMMARY

Leo is unique and typical at the same time. As his mom so eloquently wrote, his parents didn't think anyone but the two of them would ever understand him. He has his own individual traits and lovable qualities. But Leo is also similar to other children who profit from intervention that blends DTI and Incidental Intervention. He had strong entry skills in some areas, but had significant challenges in others. Most noteworthy was his compulsive fixation on his two toy animals that interfered with nearly all other activities. A strategy of teaching him to gradually give up control over the toy animals was successful. His case also illustrates the importance of therapy intensity. He was progressing slowly for the first 6 months. When his parents decided to increase therapy intensity to 30–35 hours per week and integrate Incidental Teaching with DTI, the rate of his skill acquisition greatly increased. As it progresses, Leo's therapy will increasingly be embedded in peer contexts so that his communication and social skills prepare him for successful school transition with typical peers.

REFERENCES

Berkeley, G. (2009). *A treatise concerning principles of human knowledge. Introduction, # 7.* Retrieved June 29, 2009, from Project Gutenberg, EBook #4723. (Original work published 1710)

Cowan R.J.C., & Allen, K.D. (2007). Using naturalistic procedures to enhance learning in individuals with autism: A focus on generalized teaching within the school setting. *Psychology in the Schools, 44*(7), 701–716.

Hart, B., & Risley, T. (1982). *How to use incidental teaching for elaborating language.* Austin, TX: PRO-ED.

Koegel, R.I., & Frea, W.D. (1993). Treatment of social behavior in autism through the modification of pivotal social skills. *Journal of Applied Behavior Analysis, 26*(3), 369–377.

Leaf, R., McEachin, J.J., & Harsh, J D. (1999). *A work in progress: Behavior management strategies and a curriculum for intensive behavioral treatment of autism.* New York: DRL Books.

Maurice, C., Green, G., & Luce, S.C. (1996). *Behavioral intervention for young children with autism: A manual for parents and professionals.* Austin, TX: PRO-ED.

McGee, G.G., & Daly, T. (2007). Incidental teaching of age-appropriate social phrases to children with autism. *Research & Practice for Persons with Severe Disabilities, 32*(2), 112–123.

McGee, G.G., Almeida, M.C., Sulzer-Azaroff, B., & Feldman, R.S. (1992). Promoting reciprocal interactions via peer incidental teaching. *Journal of Applied Behavior Analysis, 25,* 117–126.

McGee, G.G., Krantz, P.J., Mason, D., & McClannahan, L.E. (1983). A modified incidental-teaching procedure for autistic youth: Acquisition and generalization of receptive object labels. *Journal of Applied Behavior Analysis, 16*(3), 329–338.

McGee, G.G., Krantz, P.J., & McClannahan, L.E. (1985). The facilitative effects of incidental teaching on preposition use by autistic children. *Journal of Applied Behavior Analysis, 18*(1), 17.

Partington, J.W. (2007). *Assessment of basic language and learning skills-revised (ABLLS-R).* Walnut Creek, CA: The Behavior Analysts.

Prizant, B.M., & Wetherby, A.M. (1998). Understanding the continuum of discrete-trial traditional behavioral to social-pragmatic developmental approaches in communication enhancement for young children with autism/PDD. *Seminars in Speech and Language, 19*(4), 329–352.
Seuss, Dr. (1960). *Green eggs and ham.* New York: Random House.

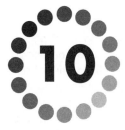

10 Blended Interventions for Children with Moderate Symptoms and Intellectual Delay

with Patti L. Dropik and Lisa M. Barsness

"It should be noted that children at play are not playing about; their games should be seen as their most serious-minded activity."

—Michel de Montaigne, *Essays* (1575)

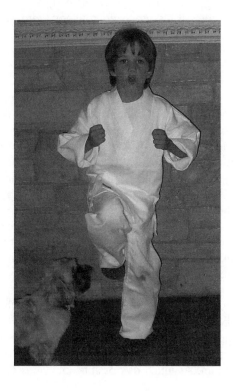

● ● ● ● ● ● ● ● ● ●

INTRODUCTION: BLAKE

In 2010, Blake was an attractive, russet-haired 7-year-old boy who most people thought was "just a regular kid" who was a little quirky at times. He had an engaging smile, with dimples in his cheeks and sparkling brown eyes. His theatrical gestures and the goofy things he did invariably got a laugh from people around him. Blake was well liked by everyone, including his typical peers and teachers at school. He attended a small private school for typically developing children his age. Blake's mom, Emily, had an M.B.A. and was an accountant and controller for a small start-up company. Until Blake was 6, Emily had been a stay-at-home mom working with Blake and overseeing his intervention. Blake's dad was self-employed as a private commercial building contractor. His 17-year-old sister, Ashley, was attending college. The family lived in a spacious home in a rural exurban area west of Minneapolis. A sister and brother-in-law who helped with Blake's child care lived nearby, and their two sons provided wonderful playmates for Blake.

To look at Blake's family then, you would never have guessed that the family had been in crisis over Blake's autism diagnosis 5 years earlier. Testing at that time suggested he had cognitive developmental delays, significant receptive-expressive language disorder, and Autistic Disorder. Emily had recognized something was different about Blake from a very early age, even before the official diagnosis. She had read extensively and was convinced he had autism. Blake was born with low muscle tone, spasticity in his neck from an unusual posture in her uterus before birth, and atypical leg positioning when seated. He underwent 2 years of physical therapy to overcome his physical challenges, which largely were eliminated. Blake was socially aloof and involved in a very small number of rigid play activities, such as building with Lincoln Logs, which he did repetitively with little or no imaginative play. He had daily tantrums if his preferred routines were interrupted. He had limited interest in playing with other children. His eye contact was fleeting or absent, sometimes even with his parents. He often failed to follow his parents' directions, sometimes acting as though he hadn't heard them. He used no verbal labels and engaged in little reciprocal conversation.

Shortly after his diagnosis at 2 years of age, his parents enrolled Blake in an intensive, home-based Discrete Trial Behavioral Intervention (DTBI) program. He developed important basic skills, but his rigid, inflexible routines continued as before and his tantrums persisted. With time, Blake reacted increasingly negatively to the DTBI program. When therapists arrived to begin therapy for the day, he ran away crying and screaming. Therapists and parents often found themselves placing Blake in a timeout chair to reduce his disruptive behavior so therapy could be conducted. Blake was clearly unhappy and resisted the well-meaning therapists who were trying to help him learn. His parents began exploring alternatives.

Emily and Curt sought our assistance at MEAP shortly before Blake's 4th birthday, enrolling him in our Blended Behavioral Intervention program involving a combination of naturalistic and DTBI methods. Interwoven were techniques borrowed from PRT (Koegel & Koegel, 2006) and activity-based early intervention (Pretti-Frontczak & Bricker, 2004). As of this writing, Blake has completed 3 years of Blended Intensive Early Intervention.

Intervention began with staff members establishing rapport with Blake while making few demands, learning what interested him, and developing hypotheses about what motivated him. As much as possible, activities directed toward specific therapy goals were incorporated into typical daily activities. Efforts were made to gradually broaden the array of play activities Blake enjoyed by using Incidental Intervention methods, occasionally supplemented by Discrete Trial techniques when new goals were introduced. By the end of the first year of Blended Intervention, therapy was either incidental or organized around play themes that Blake helped select. At that point, Blake rarely had meltdowns and had learned to tolerate denials of his preferred activities. As his communication skills became more complex and the range of his daily activities and play routines expanded, his positive personality traits became more obvious, including his sense of humor. His enjoyment of role-playing and theatrical acting became apparent. These were important changes that reminded us all that Blake was an intelligent, enjoyable child if helped to develop the skills and given the opportunity to display those aspects of himself.

Beginning with the summer of Blake's last year of Blended Intervention (his third year), nearly all of his activities were structured around peer play and learning with peers. He had been taught how to observe other children first, then to begin to participate in what they were doing, as a means of entering into other children's play. Over the summer his parents enrolled him in an unstructured community playground group of typically developing peers. Later in the summer he joined a structured learning program called Preschool Explorations, and finally toward the end of summer Blake joined the Under the Sea Journeys group, in which he thrived. He was described as "quite a thespian." His mother didn't tell the staff operating the programs that Blake had autism. He was accompanied part of the time by one of our therapists who assisted him in troubleshooting social situations, so it is likely they assumed he had some type of challenge. Nonetheless, his peers didn't seem aware that he was different from other children in those programs. They were told that our staff members were Blake's teachers. Prior to entering school in the fall, Blake helped implement and participate in a school thematic intervention activity (described later) that helped prepare him for what to expect and to acquire the necessary skills to negotiate typical school situations.

● ● ● ● ● ● ● ● ● ●

THERAPY PRINCIPLES AND ASSUMPTIONS

Roots in Incidental and Milieu Language Intervention Plus Activity-Based Intervention

Blended Interventions are based on ABA principles integrated with naturalistic teaching strategies and activity-based early intervention. *Incidental Teaching* refers to the use of normally occurring situations in a child's daily activities and use of the child's interest to promote learning (Hart & Risley, 1975). Incidental Teaching has been used for both social skills as well as language intervention (Koegel & Frea, 1993; McGee, Almeida, Sulzer-Azaroff, & Feldman, 1992). As much as possible, the activity is selected by the child (Hart & Risley, 1975), with the caregiver following the child's lead. Incidental Teaching strategies are especially effective in facilitating carryover across adult caregivers and settings.

Among other early intervention strategies, *activity-based intervention* (ABI; Pretti-Frontczak & Bricker, 2004) is widely accepted within the preschool/early intervention community. The approach grows out of constructivist developmental theory (Pretti-Frontczak & Bricker, 2004). In Blended Interventions, some of the strategies employed in activity-based early intervention are combined with Behavioral Incidental Teaching, such as PRT (Koegel & Koegel, 2006).

Embedding "Trials" within Thematic Activities

For many children with moderate to higher functioning autism, organizing intervention activities around thematic activities—such as eating at a restaurant, a visit to the doctor's office, shopping at the supermarket, or going to the library—can create the context within which specific skills can be taught. For example, Blake participated in a restaurant thematic activity that included three roles—the waiter, cashier, and customer—involving nine different types of activities from three people's perspectives. Note that embedded within each interactive exchange for the three roles, the therapist encourages several flexible responses from Blake to varying situational cues that function as learning "trials," though they are not in the context of a Discrete Trial format.

Figure 10.1 shows the recording sheet from Blake's restaurant thematic activity used to teach behavior associated with the waiter's perspective. This recording sheet was used to track his performance on various subgoals within this Incidental Intervention activity.

Learning Is Incremental and by Leaps and Bounds

Some intervention is accomplished in the context of games or ongoing play. For example, early in Blake's intervention he was taught to label items based on the description of their features. The therapist would say, "I'm thinking of something with four legs and a tail that barks. What is it?" His progress was slow initially, but then accelerated to the goal of correctly labeling at least 25 items. Later, with only a few repetitions of a scenario, correct responses occurred much more rapidly. For example, Blake was being taught to more accurately monitor social cues (e.g., body language, posture, gestures, tone of voice). He was asked to identify the emotion being expressed and explain what action he could take to respond to the person's feelings. Blake's baseline was 10% correct at the beginning of the month, rising to 50% by the end of the month, reaching 100% correct in 2 months. More important, he generalized to spontaneous natural situations 90% of the time within 2 months.

Capitalizing on the Child's Interests and Aptitudes

An essential element of making Blended Intervention effective is building on a child's interests, skills, and natural aptitudes. Another parent was interested in involving her son, Jay, in sports, and decided to try T-ball. Unfortunately, Jay had no understanding of the game other than batting the ball. He had an awkward gait, and it was difficult for him to run the bases without falling or running so slowly that he was always called out. Involving Jay in a sport would have been more successful if his parents had been guided by Jay's interests and skill level. He enjoyed playing indoor games like nine-pins, which did not involve the complex rules of a team competitive sport and didn't require running. Also, nine-pins' pacing was determined by Jay rather than the adult leading the T-ball game.

Structured Learning Opportunities

Blended Interventions differ from Incidental Teaching Interventions in that the adult loosely structures the learning opportunities rather than waiting for the child to "take the lead." For example, one day Blake's therapist Jennifer said, "I have a surprise toy

Thematic Activity

Child's name: ___Blake_____

Parent name(s): ___Emily_____

Instructions: Record "+": independent; "P": staff prompt; "−": did not use appropriate play action and/or language.

	Date: 6/16	Date: 6/30	Date: 7/2	Date: 7/6	Date: 7/14	Date: 7/21	Date: 7/28	Date: 8/5	Date: 8/12
Role 1: Waiter/waitress									
1. Host activities (score actions)									
Score language: *Welcome to SpongeBob Restaurant. Would you like to sit at a booth or a table? How many people are eating with you? My name is Blake and I'll be your waiter. Follow me to your table.*	−	−	−	P	P	−	P	P	+
2. Take order (score actions)									
Score language: *Today's special is tomato (or chicken noodle) soup. When do you want your drink? Your dessert? How would you like that? What side orders do you want? The chicken comes with a salad. I'll take your menu. It will be 10 minutes to cook your food. I'll give your order to the chef.*	−	P	P	−	P	P	+	+	+
3. Make/bring food (score actions)									
Score language: *Be careful, it's hot. Here's your dinner, beverage, dessert. Enjoy your meal. When do you want your bill? How does your dinner taste? Is there anything else you need?*	−	−	−	P	P	−	P	+	+
4. Bring bill (score actions)									
Score language: *Here's your bill. You can pay when you finish eating. Pay at the cash register. Leave your money on the table.*	P	P	P	P	+	+	+	+	+

Figure 10.1. Blake's restaurant Thematic Activity sheet, recording teaching behavior associated with two perspective-taking roles with specific goals for each, under specified stimulus conditions.

(continued)

Thematic Activity *(continued)*

Instructions: Record "+": independent, "P"; staff prompt; "−": did not use appropriate play action and/or language.

Role 2: Cashier	Date: 6/16	Date: 6/30	Date: 7/2	Date: 7/6	Date: 7/14	Date: 7/21	Date: 7/28	Date: 8/5	Date: 8/12
1. Go up to customer. Offer him or her the bill. (score actions)									
Score language: *Your bill is 10 dollars. Thank you for eating at SpongeBob Restaurant. Come back to eat here again.*	−	P	−	P	P	P	P	P	P

Instructions: Record "+": independent, "P": staff prompt; "−": did not use appropriate play action and/or language.

Role 3: Customer	Date: 6/16	Date: 6/30	Date: 7/2	Date: 7/6	Date: 7/14	Date: 7/21	Date: 7/28	Date: 8/5	Date: 8/12
1. Enter restaurant. Wait to be seated. Follow host's instructions. (score actions)									
Score language: *I would like a table for three. Can I sit by a window? My friends and I are starving, will you seat us?*	−	−	P	P	P	+	+	+	+
2. Give order (score actions)									
Score language: *What do you recommend? Does the soup taste good? I'll have a small, medium, large lemonade. I want a lot of fries and a little bit of ketchup. Hold the salt. For dessert I'll have ice cream. We will share dessert; could you bring us an extra spoon? When will our food be ready?*	−	−	−	−	P	−	P	P	+

	Date: 6/16	Date: 6/30	Date: 7/2	Date: 7/6	Date: 7/14	Date: 7/21	Date: 7/28	Date: 8/5	Date: 8/12
3. Thank waiter/waitress. Eat food. (score actions)									
Score language: *Thank you for bringing my food. This chicken looks and smells delicious. Ouch! This coffee is too hot! I need another napkin. Excuse me, could I have a refill of my juice?*	−	−	P	−	P	P	P	+	+
4. Ask where to pay. Pay cashier. (score actions)									
Score language: *The food was very good. Could you tell me where I take my bill? Thank you. Have a nice day!*	−	−	−	P	P	+	+	+	+

bag. Put your hand in and feel one of the toys with your hand and tell me how the toy feels. I'll try to guess what it is." The purpose of this activity was to give Blake practice in developing descriptive vocabulary in a motivating context.

Blake said, "It's got wheels and drives on roads."

Jennifer guessed, "It's an airplane!"

"No," Blake laughed. "Airplanes don't drive on roads."

"Hmm, let's see, it must be a car," Jennifer said.

"Right!" Blake shouted, and then said, "OK, it's your turn."

Jennifer put her hand in the bag and described a dog. This activity is flexible and unpredictable, but structured so that a range of possibilities can be anticipated.

Thematic activities are partially structured by the caregiver, but the child also has a significant role in selecting what will be done. When Blake chooses "Going to the Doctor" as the theme, he is asked to decide what materials they will need to play that activity. In doing so, he is taught to think analytically and develop vocabulary related to going to the doctor (e.g., "blood pressure thing," "heart listening thing," "injection thing," "x-ray"). He is asked whether he wants to be the doctor or patient first, and he usually chooses the role of doctor. That provides a range of activities he can practice and also helps him learn the doctor's perspective. Jennifer wiggles when Blake tries to take her blood pressure with the cuff. She says, "What does the doctor think?" "He wants her to sit still so he can take her blood pressure." When Jennifer asks, "What does the doctor say to the patient?" Blake replies, "Okay girl, sit still so I can take your blood pressure." Jennifer tries not to laugh.

Overcoming Compulsive Routines

Nearly all children on the autism spectrum have some highly preferred activities into which they lapse if nothing else is occupying their attention. For some, it is watching preferred DVDs. For others, it is rocking and visual self-stimulation. Several years ago I worked with a preschooler with autism who was obsessed with Thomas the Tank Engine. His father had installed an elaborate electric train set in the family room on which the boy perseverated. He constantly wanted to play with the train set and had meltdowns if anyone else attempted to touch the train.

Blake's obsessive-compulsive routines involved talking about and drawing pictures of *Goosebumps*, R.L. Stine's series of children's horror fiction novellas that have spun off board games, videos, and other related products. Blake was obsessed with *Goosebumps*; incessantly talking about the characters and drawing pictures of goosebumps. Reducing Blake's preoccupation with *Goosebumps* involved increasing his interest in other games and fictional characters, while simultaneously limiting his time spent involved with Goosebumps-related activities. He was able to contract for 5 minutes at the end of each therapy shift during which he could look at *Goosebumps* books or draw *Goosebumps* characters. During these periods no one talked with him or expressed interest in what he was doing. The goal was to avoid inadvertently reinforcing his behavior related to Goosebumps activities. Over several months his preoccupation with *Goosebumps* waned and eventually receded into the background.

Capitalizing on Social Interest

Within a year of beginning Blended Intervention, Blake began showing interest in other children. He watched them and seemed to want to play with them but had no idea how to enter into their play. In the beginning he would approach another child and say something like "Hey, Boy, let's play cars" and try to interest the other child in his toy car. Needless to say, this wasn't very effective. The other child, who was engaged in a different activity, usually walked away. Blake seldom used people's names. The fact that he was socially interested meant there was a natural motivator for learning new social skills (Jahr, Eldevik, & Eikeseth, 2000). Therapists began by encouraging Blake to learn the names of children with whom he regularly interacted, and later to address them by name. Figure 10.2 shows Blake's receptive and expressive name use in an unstructured play group (Neighborhood Playground Group), in a structured program involving the same children on each occasion (Preschool Explorations), and in a summer theater group (Sea Journeys). Though his baseline recognition of children's names was zero in June, within a month he was correctly identifying and addressing children by names 90% to 100% of the time. When he entered the summer theater group, where he knew none of the children's names, his baseline was zero, but within a week he had exceeded 80% correct. His expressive name use was nearly 100% until a new group of children entered the group, when it dropped considerably. In fall when he entered school, he soon learned all of the children's names and addressed his classmates by their names.

Maintaining Intensity in Natural Settings

Intervention intensity is important in achieving therapy goals. In DTI, intervention intensity is determined largely by therapists or the teacher through pacing of trials and activities, which means it is relatively easy to maintain sufficient intensity. In both Blended and Incidental Intervention, intensity depends considerably on the child's in-

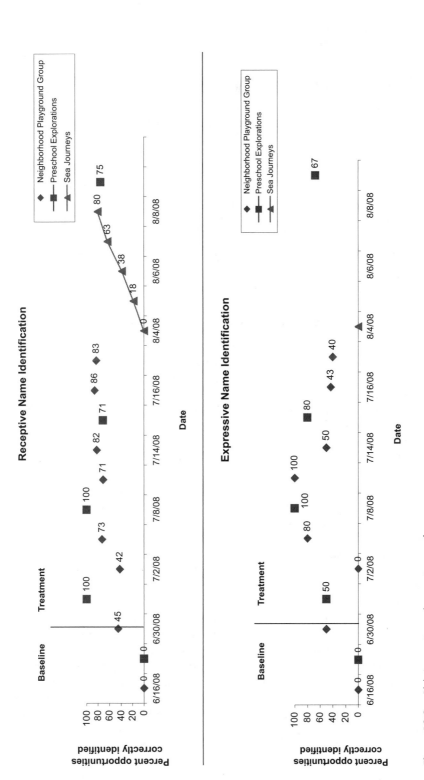

Figure 10.2. Blake's receptive and expressive use of peer names.

terests and willingness to participate with minimal prompting and take the lead. It is somewhat easier to maintain sufficient therapy intensity in Blended Intervention settings than in totally Incidental Interventions, because there is more predictability of intervention opportunities.

Most of the activities from which the child chooses are made available by the therapist. For example, "Should we play 'What Am I Feeling,' Blake?" says Jennifer, "or should we play, 'I See?'" Blake chooses, "What Am I Feeling," and waits for Jennifer's signal. Jennifer crosses her arms across her chest and frowns. Blake laughs. "You're mad," Blake says. "Now it's your turn. Show me how you are feeling," Jennifer says to Blake. Blake smiles broadly, and Jennifer says, "I think you are happy." "Right," Blake replies. Having learned to discriminate others' feelings, the next step involved teaching him appropriate responses depending on another person's emotions (Schrandt, Townsend, & Poulson, 2009).

We encourage therapy staff to prepare a "cheat sheet" before their therapy sessions, which they place on a clipboard, listing sequential opportunities within activities to embed interventions addressing individualized treatment plan goals. In some less structured situations, social opportunities are less predictable. Each week therapy staff members are asked to record the number of activities addressing individualized treatment plan goals for a given session, using a tally counter attached to their waistband. If the numbers begin to decline over weeks, staff members meet and brainstorm methods for ensuring adequate therapy intensity.

Create and Maintain Independent Creative Activities

A goal of Blended Intervention is to provide children with the skills to independently occupy themselves in creative, appropriately stimulating activities. This involves several individual steps that, when combined, lead a child to be capable of occupying him- or herself for an extended time interval (e.g., 20–30 minutes). For example, Zachary, who was 3½ years old, tended to lapse into nonfunctional self-stimulatory activities if he wasn't busy with a constructive pursuit. His therapist taught him how to play with five different interesting toys, one at a time, and then combined them using a visual schedule. The toys included a complex shape sorter, a jigsaw puzzle, a Lego set, and two other activities. Zachary was taught to use each toy, one at a time. Then he was taught how to use a visual schedule to guide him from one activity to the next. Finally, all five games or toys were presented sequentially on a visual schedule. He only needed a prompt at the beginning, such as, "Zachary, look at your schedule." Then, he would play with each game or toy until it had been completed, put it away, and take out the next toy, until he had played with all five toys. That usually required 15–20 minutes of constructively spent activity. This was not only good for Zachary but also helpful to his parents, who were now able to occupy him in positive ways without constant prompts and attention.

A similar strategy was used with Blake, except that he was taught to create his own hand-printed schedule at the beginning of each session, selecting from a much wider array of choices. He had in the past used a visual schedule when he first began EIBI, as well as in school, so he was familiar with schedules. At home, he would be prompted to look at his schedule, and then for the next half hour he would occupy himself constructively with a series of play activities of his own choosing, such as reading a book to his stuffed animals, Play-Doh, cars, and so forth. His self-selected activities varied somewhat from day to day, depending on his mood and interest. Eventually he learned to create his plan of activities on his own without prompting.

Generalizing to Natural Family Settings

A major reason for using Blended Interventions is that transfer of skills from a therapy situation to naturally occurring daily routines is greatly facilitated. Once Blake learned to create his own list of activities with which to occupy himself, when his parents were busy with something else such as meal preparation, they could simply say, "Blake, look at your schedule," which led him to undertake several appropriate, typical activities in which any child his age might engage.

Thematic activities are specifically selected because they include elements that are the same as daily routine activities, like going shopping or to the doctor's office, which facilitates transfer of learned skills. After Blake had practiced the restaurant theme, his family went out to dinner at a restaurant and Blake was indistinguishable from other kids his age at the restaurant. He read the menu, ordered his own food, and he even asked the waiter what kinds of spices were in the spaghetti sauce.

ROOTS IN APPLIED BEHAVIOR ANALYSIS PRINCIPLES

Not long ago, a behavior analyst colleague observed one of our therapists who was using a Blended Intervention strategy in working with a child with autism, and he asked the therapist if she was conducting play therapy (i.e., experiential, attachment-based or psychodynamic treatment built around children's play; Schaefer & Kaduson, 2006). It is easy to make this mistake if one isn't aware of what to look for in the adult–child interactions. Blended Interventions are based on ABA principles (Cooper, Heron, & Heward, 2007) but incorporate techniques from milieu language intervention and activity-based early intervention. Teachers' or therapists' comments or requests (e.g., "I wonder what we should do next?"), along with the presence of natural play materials (Play-Doh containers and felt-tip pens and colored paper are on the table before the child), provide the stimuli that set the occasion for the child's responses. Reinforcing consequences are less often something to eat or drink than in DTI, but edibles are included occasionally if the child contracts for such a reward for achieving what he or she set out to accomplish (e.g., "Can I have a fruit roll-up when I finish the puzzle?"). Reinforcing consequences are typically natural activities or events, like going out to play when toys have been put away, and nearly always incorporate positive comments (e.g., "Wow, that was terrific!") or "high fives." Among the most common reinforcing consequences is access to a preferred activity, which may be socializing with the therapist or a peer (e.g., "horseback rides" on the caregiver's back, playing a game with a peer).

Blended Behavioral Intervention is an outgrowth of Incidental Teaching and milieu language intervention that employs 1) language teaching that follows the child's interest, 2) use of multiple, naturally occurring examples, 3) explicit prompts for the child to use language, 4) the use of natural consequences to reinforce the child's verbal behavior, and 5) the use of embedded naturalistic language teaching strategies in the ongoing interactions between parent, therapist, or teacher and the child (Kaiser, Yoder, & Keetz, 1992; Koegel, Vernon, & Koegel, 2009). Participating in an activity in which the child is already interested makes learning or therapy much more effective and enjoyable for the child. Using naturally occurring situations and consequences ensures generalization. Embedding intervention in ongoing child–parent interactions capitalizes upon the natural stimulus-response-reinforcement relations that promote learning and maintain behavior in everyday life.

Monitoring Child Progress

Like DTI, Blended Interventions require that data are collected regularly as the basis for determining whether the intervention is effective. In DTI, correct or incorrect responses are often collected on a trial-by-trial basis. Because there are generally no trials in Blended Interventions, several other strategies are used to monitor child progress. Periodic probes are conducted in which specific skills are tested over several inserted trials (e.g., whether the child correctly identifies emotions based on facial expressions). An alternative is to record spontaneously occurring events, such as whether the child with ASD establishes eye contact when he or she attempts to recruit a peer's attention during free play. The disadvantage of this approach is that the number of spontaneous instances may be very small and may vary widely from day to day, depending on what is being evaluated. In thematic activities, often there are *specific kinds of responses* that are appropriate in a given situation that can be recorded as occurring or not occurring, or as only occurring with prompting. If Blake is playing the role of the waiter in a restaurant, did he remember to offer the customer a menu? In some instances, natural language samples are also taken to determine complexity of spoken language under specific circumstances.

In Figure 10.3, *mean length of utterance* (MLU) is a measure of language complexity in children. A *morpheme* is any word or word part that conveys meaning and cannot be divided into smaller elements that also can convey meaning. A higher MLU is taken to indicate a higher level of language competence. It is calculated in morphemes or in words by dividing the number of morphemes or words by the total number of utterances, with an *utterance* defined as a sequence of words preceded and followed by change of turn in a conversation. Miller and Chapman (1981) reported that the average growth of morphemes is 1.2 per year for typical preschool children. Figure 10.3 shows that Blake's MLUs increased by 0.45 and the number of words grew by 0.25 in 3 months, which, prorated over a year would be an increase of 1.0 MLUs for the year—reasonable language growth.

Setting: Home, School, and Community

Whereas DTI usually takes place at home or at school, and often in a single room (at least in the beginning), by definition, Blended Interventions can occur in the backyard, on the playground at school, in the park, at the library, and so on. Most places the child typically spends her or his time are appropriate for Blended Intervention, unless the associated stimuli are too distracting or overwhelming (e.g., at the water park, while

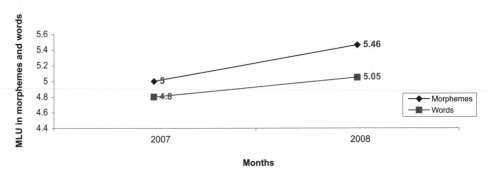

Figure 10.3. Growth of Blake's language complexity as measured by increase in mean length of utterance over 4 months from November 2007 to February 2008.

watching a parade). Blended Intervention is started at home in various rooms in the house and then soon transfers to outdoor locations adjacent to the home. Next, more controlled community settings, such as the library or park, are included as venues, and finally more crowded, unpredictable settings are included, such as shopping malls. Thematic activities are done at home or sometimes at a peer's home as spontaneous social skills are targeted for intervention. At times, we work with the same child at home, for example, in the morning, and for part of the afternoon in preschool focusing on social skills to promote generalization of skills across settings and people (McGrath, Bosch, Sullivan, & Fuqua, 2003).

Theme-Based Materials

The main difference between materials used in Blended Intervention and DTI is greater complexity and variability among Blended Intervention materials (see Chapter 8). Children involved in Blended Intervention typically have more language than those in DTI, so as a result, more activities involving printing, reading, and listening to stories, or more complex spoken communications are incorporated. Instead of depending primarily on a small number of simple action toys or closed-ended activities such as form puzzles, as is done in DTI, many more open-ended activities are used, such as arts and crafts and creative play activities, including costumes for dress-up role playing. It is often useful to ask the child to help create materials used in thematic activities, in part because it requires him or her to think about aspects of the situations that will be role-played (e.g., for a library theme: books, CDs, bookshelves, wall clock, library card, and check out scanner). If the child makes the materials himself of herself, he or she is more likely to be interested in the activity and will be more actively involved in using appropriate vocabulary to discuss the venue.

Assessment

Blake's Baseline Assessment of Basic Language and Learning Skills-Revised

At the beginning of Blended Intervention, Blake exhibited strong skills in cooperation, imitation, and vocal imitation, shown in his ABLLS-R (Figure 10.4). He also had strengths in receptive and expressive communication. Blake had deficits in making requests, labeling, and responding to more complex aspects of spoken communication (intraverbals).

Sample Verbal Behavior Milestones Assessment and Placement Program

Figure 10.5 shows a baseline VB-MAPP system profile for Robin, a child similar to Blake, kindly provided by Dr. Mark Sundberg (2008). Note that Robin's entry skills at 2 years of age were limited to Level 1, corresponding to birth to 18 months of age for a typically developing child. Robin's strengths are in listening (receptive language), matching and sorting, play, and imitation, all prerequisites to more complex skills. Like the ABLLS, the VB-MAPP is a criterion-referenced assessment and does not make it possible to compare performance against standard norms of typically developing children (percentiles), but it does make it possible to design interventions based on specific existing and lacking skills. The VB-MAPP manual provides intervention suggestions for each skill.

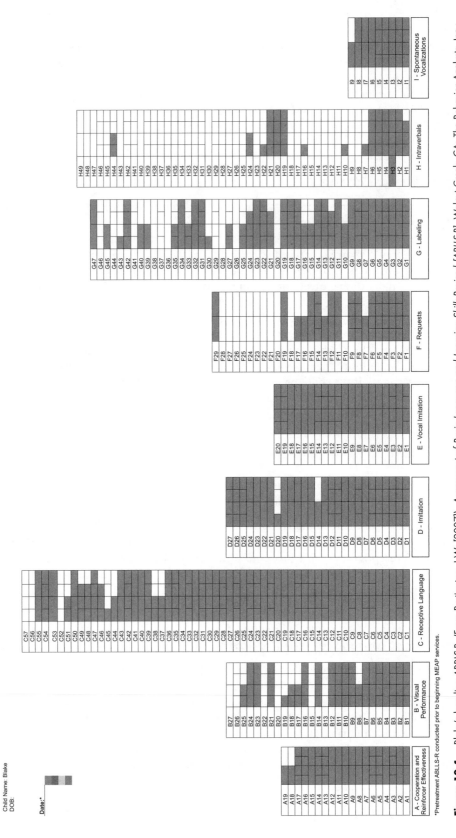

Figure 10.4. Blake's baseline ABBLS-R. (From Partington, J.W. [2007]). *Assessment of Basic Language and Learning Skills-Revised [ABLLS-R].* Walnut Creek, CA: The Behavior Analysts, Inc.; adapted by permission.)

Child's name:	Robin				
Date of birth:	6/7/2006				
Age of testing:	1	3.4	2	3	4

Key:	Score	Date	Color	Test
1st test:	12.5	10/14/09		TT
2nd test:				
3rd test:				
4th test:				

LEVEL 3

Mand	Tact	Listener	VP/MTS	Play	Social	Reading	Writing	LRFFC	IV	Group	Ling	Math

LEVEL 2

Mand	Tact	Listener	VP/MTS	Play	Social	Reading	Echoic	LRFFC	IV	Group	Ling

LEVEL 1

Mand	Tact	Listener	VP/MTS	Play	Social	Reading	Echoic	Vocal

Figure 10.5. Sample Verbal Behavior Milestones Assessment and Placement Program system profile. (From Sundberg, M.L. [2008]. *Verbal behavior milestones assessment and placement program [VB-MAPP]*. Concord, CA: Advancements in Verbal Behavior Press; reprinted by permission.)

Beginning Therapy

As with DTI, Blended Intervention is usually begun in a single comfortable location, such as a family room or the child's bedroom. As soon as rapport has been established as in DTI (Chapter 7), therapy is extended to other rooms in the house, as long as they are not too distracting (e.g., home theater or multimedia rooms). If the child chooses to move from one room to another over the course of intervention, generally the therapist follows and continues intervention in the new location. Often the rapport-building process proceeds somewhat more rapidly than in DTI, but 4–6 weeks of gradually increasing weekly intervention hours and slowly introducing demands is typical. If a child shows signs of resistance, no new activities are added for several days or a week, and the rate of prompts per session is decreased. Once the child's demeanor and behavior indicates she or he is happily participating, new activities are introduced according to her or his IEP or individualized treatment plan. Therapists and teachers often present two or three choices of activities during each session, permitting the child to choose. If the child suggests another activity, as long as it is possible to embed activities toward the treatment plan goals in the endeavor, it is included (see Figure 10.6). By the end of 6 weeks, 20–30 hours per week of intervention is occurring, and by the end of the first quarter, usually the child's intervention is going smoothly and behavioral challenges are markedly waning or have ceased.

● ● ● ● ● ● ● ● ● ●

BLAKE: A CHILD WHO THRIVED ON BLENDED INTERVENTION

Blake appeared on the surface to be much like other children his age, but on closer examination, he displayed a variety of behavioral characteristics that distinguished him from his typically developing peers. His interests were very limited, he had frequent tantrums, and lacked basic communication and social skills. However, he showed social interest and had a very actively involved family that participated in his intervention. The resulting changes in Blake's ability to function similar to typical peers were dramatic.

Blake at Baseline

When Blake was evaluated at age 2, his physical examination revealed he was of average height and weight with normal hearing and vision. His intellectual functioning had been in the low average range and his autism diagnostic testing produced a score in the Autistic Disorder range. During our intake assessment at our clinic 2 years later, Blake exhibited little eye contact with our staff, one of whom was seated on the floor next to where he was playing with a toy car. He looked up periodically to see what the adults were doing but did not show interest in interacting with adults. During an initial home visit, Blake was alert and talking a great deal, mostly to himself and sometimes to his mother, though he seldom appeared to respond to what she said in reply. He was seated on the floor playing with Lincoln Logs. He had a very alert facial expression. He occasionally looked up when someone spoke to him, but not always. When a staff member attempted to switch from Lincoln Logs to another game, he began whining and held on to the Lincoln Logs so they couldn't be taken away, although no one had threatened to put them away. When intervention was first begun, his mother asked that we continue to use time out in his chair in the corridor to control his whining, which occurred daily. She had developed a strategy of warning him once by saying "Absolutely not!" in a stern voice, and if that did not stop his whining he was led to the time-out chair. He occasionally hit during those episodes, but that was infrequent.

It was obvious from the outset that Blake was very capable, but his intolerance for trying new activities and his lack of social interest and poor communication skills severely limited his opportunities. First goals were built around developing pivotal skills that would have wide ramifications throughout his daily life. Goals included improved eye contact, greeting people and returning greetings, and increased positive response to social overtures by peers.

Blake's Individualized Treatment Plan

Figure 10.6 shows Blake's individualized treatment plan goals early during intervention. Objectives are divided into communication, socialization, and repetitive behavior and fixed interests.

Treatment Goals and Objectives:

Child's name: __Blake_____ Date of birth: _____

Parent(s) name(s): __Emily_____

I. Communication

Long-term goal	**1. Describes objects and people using phrases and sentences**		
Short-term goal	When requested, Blake will describe novel, yet familiar, objects and people using phrases and/or sentences that include at least 3 varied descriptors for target with no visual stimuli across 3 consecutive "yes" probes, 2 staff, and at least 1 parent or caregiver.		
Strategies/teaching methods	When asked to describe an object/person/location/event, the practitioner or parent will provide Blake with a verbal model of at least 3 descriptors. Practitioners/parents will fade prompts and provide differential reinforcement for independent, correct responses.		
Date introduced	3/11/08	Projected mastery date	9/23/08

Long-term goal	**2. Similarities and differences**		
Short-term goal	When requested, Blake will identify similarities and differences between at least 3 novel exemplars of objects/people/locations and events across 3 consecutive "yes" probes, 2 staff, and 1 parent or caregiver.		
Strategies/teaching methods	When asked to verbally identify similarities and differences between objects/people/locations or events, the practitioner or parent will provide Blake with a model and may use visual cues to prompt the correct response. Practitioners/parents will fade prompts and provide differential reinforcement for independent, correct responses.		
Date introduced	7/23/08	Projected mastery date	11/23/08

Long-term goal	**3. Maintains topic in conversation**		
Short-term goal	Blake will maintain a play episode on topic for at least 5 minutes for 5 different themes by using appropriate language for play theme when playing with a single peer as assessed during at least 80% of intervals across 2 consecutive probes.		

Figure 10.6. Blake's individualized treatment plan illustrating goals in each core symptom area (communication, socialization, and restricted and repetitive behavior) as well as family skills goals.

(continued)

Treatment Goals and Objectives *(continued)*

Strategies/treatment methods	The practitioner/parent will model on topic language during themed play units, picture book reading, and functional daily living contexts. Practitioners/parents will use verbal models and open-ended questions to prompt Blake to use appropriate play language that is on topic and not related to a perseverative interest/behavior such as monsters, drawing, or building with blocks. Prompts will be faded gradually and differential reinforcement will be provided for spontaneous imitation and independent maintenance of topic with language.		
Date introduced	4/8/08	Projected mastery date	11/23/08

Long-term Goal	**4. Attends and listens to partner responses to Blake's verbal initiations**		
Short-term goal	When Blake verbally initiates a question or statement directed to practitioner/parent and peer, he will practice appropriate listening behaviors—wait for and attend to partner's response—80% of opportunities across at least 2 contexts and 2 days.		
Strategies/treatment	When Blake initiates verbally to parent/practitioner or peer, practitioner will prompt Blake to demonstrate appropriate listening behavior (e.g., waiting, looking at partner, facing partner, etc.). Prompts will be faded gradually and differential reinforcement will be provided for spontaneous and independent waiting/attending responses.		
Date introduced	8/23/08	Projected mastery date	11/23/08

II. Socialization

Long-term goal	**5. Develop and increase sequenced play actions across a variety of topics**		
Short-term goal methods	Blake will increase number of play sequences/actions on a theme by 50% of play exchanges demonstrated at baseline with practitioner, peer during home peer play session.		
Strategies/treatment methods	Blake or the practitioner/parent will initiate a play interaction. Blake will sequence play actions on a theme to maintain play interaction. Practitioner/parents will provide Blake with prompts to chain multiple play actions and gradually fade prompts while providing differential reinforcement for independently sequenced play actions.		
Date introduced	3/11/08	Projected mastery date	11/23/08

Long-term goal	**6. Maintains topic with play actions**		
Short-term goal	Blake will maintain a play episode on topic for at least 5 minutes for 5 different themes by performing play actions that are on topic with play theme when playing with single peer as assessed during at least 80% of intervals across 2 consecutive probes.		
Strategies/treatment methods	The practitioner/parent will provide Blake with models of on-topic play actions during themed play units, picture book reading, and functional daily living contexts. Practitioners/parents will use verbal and nonverbal models to prompt Blake to use appropriate play actions that are on topic and not related to a perseverative interest/behavior such as monsters, drawing, or building with blocks. Prompts will be faded gradually and differential reinforcement will be provided for spontaneous imitation and independent maintenance of topic with play.		
Date introduced	4/8/08	Projected mastery date	11/23/08

III. Restricted and Repetitive Behavior Goals

Long-term Goal	**7. Decrease restricted, stereotyped pattern of behavior**		
Short-term Goal	Blake will reduce frequency of stereotyped restricted behaviors such as rigidity with block building and perseverative drawing by 80% of the average frequency during baseline assessment.		
Strategies/treatment methods	A functional assessment will be conducted to assess the variables surrounding the behavior. Evidence-based treatment strategies will be matched to the function of the behavior. Differential reinforcement of appropriate, functional block play and drawing and/or alternative activities is one technique that may be utilized.		
Date introduced	8/1/08	Projected mastery date	11/23/08
Implemented by	Mental health professionals, practitioners, and parents	Medically necessary?	Yes
Date introduced	6/23/08	Projected mastery date	11/23/08

Embedding Individualized Treatment Plan Goal Activities within Thematic Play

Figure 10.7 shows steps for embedding of Blake's individualized treatment plan goals within the restaurant thematic activity. These are more advanced goals, set after a year of Blended Intervention. This table outlines the steps required to set up the thematic activity and how to implement it. The left column indicates specific treatment plan goals and the next column provides intervention suggestions for each goal. The middle and fourth columns list anticipated concepts and vocabulary likely to arise during theme activity, and the far right column indicates how the outcomes are measured.

Contrary to the notion that naturalistic early behavioral intervention activities are a type of play therapy, meaning unstructured experiential or psychodynamic treatment, Blended Intervention thematic activities have specific materials, intervention procedures, child and caregiver expectations, goals, and measures associated with these activities.

Blake's Sample Outcomes

Figure 10.8 through Figure 10.10 show sample graphs illustrating the course of skill acquisition and expansion for Blake in several distinct individualized treatment plan goal areas. Early in intervention, Blake tended to speak in monologues, often drifting off the topic of conversation, so an early goal was to increase his ability to remain on topic. The expansion of his ability to describe things, actions, and people using appropriate vocabulary was helpful in his later social development (Figure 10.8). Later goals included the ability to effectively join in ongoing play and to monitor social cues to determine whether a listener was losing interest.

Figure 10.9 shows improvement in Blake's ability to maintain on-topic conversation within a dress-up thematic play activity. Blake exhibited increased independence with prompted appropriate conversations decreasing by over 30% and unprompted independent appropriate conversation increasing by over 50% over 3 months of therapy.

Blake's interactions with peers were initially often unsuccessful, in part because he failed to address peers by name and he often ignored his peers' interests and preferred activities. Baseline testing revealed that he seldom knew the names of children in his preschool classroom. Intervention involved first teaching him children's names receptively, and then asking him to use their names when addressing them (e.g., "Bobby, want to play cars?").

Blake's success in school depended on his ability to accurately observe what his peers were playing and to successfully join in their play. Figure 10.10 shows his progress in learning to join in ongoing peer play.

Family's Perspective: Blake

Blake was diagnosed with autism just after his second birthday. The diagnosis was not a surprise; I had noticed signs that indicated something was wrong after his first birthday. Blake was in his own world: He didn't respond to his name, didn't make eye contact, threw violent tantrums for no apparent reason, and completely ignored others around him. He also didn't like being held. The only way I could hug him is if he backed into me; he would then let me quickly hug him while he faced away

Embedded Objectives in Play Activity: *Restaurant*

Child's name: ___Blake___

Parent name(s): ___Emily___

Date: ___7/28/08___

ITP long-term/ short-term objectives	Theme concepts/ vocabulary		Assessment
1. Expresses complex meanings in functional communication contexts Blake will increase the diversity of vocabulary used to express meaning in functional communication contexts by 20% above baseline levels as assessed by number of different words used in monthly communication samples.	Practitioner will model and prompt theme vocabulary (e.g., nouns, verbs, descriptors) during theme play. I am your *waitress* and I will take your *order*. Here is your *menu*. I have to put the pizza in the oven to *bake* it. Please *pay* the *cashier* after you get your *check*. I'll *serve* you because the pizza is very *hot*.	**Nouns** *waitress/waiter* *cashier* *customer* *menu* *(customer's) order* *breakfast* *lunch* *dinner* *dessert* *fruits, vegetables, drinks* *apron* *check/bill/tip* *specials* **Verbs** *order* *bring* *cook* *bake* *serve* *clear (table/dishes)* *pay* *deliver (e.g., pizza)* *take-out* **Descriptors** *salty* *sweet* *hot* *cold* *small, medium, large* *sticky* *delicious* *hungry* *full* *empty*	Daily Play Log Language sampling— number of different words

Figure 10.7. Steps for embedding Blake's individualized treatment plan goals within a typical thematic activity.

(continued)

Embedded Objectives in Play Activity: Restaurant *(continued)*

ITP long-term/ short-term objectives	Language structures	Theme concepts/ vocabulary	Assessment
2. Expresses complex meanings in functional communication contexts Blake will increase the length/complexity of his utterances by 1 word on average by using descriptors, prepositional phrases, simple compound nouns/ verbs/phrases and early conditional clauses (*before, after, if, when, because, so*) when requesting, as assessed by monthly spontaneous communication samples.	Practitioner will recast (model correct structure) Blake's language during play set up, figurine, and role play. (See expanded manding hand-out.) I am your waitress *and* I will take your order. Here is your menu. I have to put the pizza in the oven to bake it. Please pay the cashier after you get your check.	Compound nouns, verbs, phrases (conjoin nouns, verbs, phrases using *and*) Prepositional phrases Conditional clauses (e.g., clauses that use *so, if, because, when, before, after*)	Daily Play Log Daily Data Sheet—expanded manding Language sampling (mean length of utterance)

		Examples of "wh" questions		
3. Discriminates "wh" questions (who/what/ where/ when/why) When presented with novel, developmentally appropriate "wh-" questions, Blake	Practitioner will ask "wh" questions during book reading, art/craft activity play set up, organizing, and activity roles	**Who** Who are you going to be? I'm the customer. Who takes my order? **What** What does the waitress say/do? What does the customer say/do?	**Where** Where does the waitress work? Where are the customers? Where is my apron? Order pad? Where is the restaurant? Where do you want to sit?	Daily Data Sheet

ITP long-term/ short-term objectives	Theme concepts/ vocabulary		Assessment
will respond appropriately on 80% of 5 consecutive assessments in both structured and functional contexts.	What does the cashier say/do? What does the cook say/do? What are you doing? What are you going to be, do? What is this (hold up menu or other prop)? What is this for (hold up order pad, cooking utensil)? What would you like to order?	**When** When are we going to the restaurant? When does restaurant open? When will our food be ready? When is the pizza going in the oven? **Why** Why do you need menu, order pad, and so forth? Why are you ordering chocolate ice cream? Why can't we order now?	
4. Maintains topic with language Blake will maintain a play episode for at least 5 minutes for 5 different themes by using appropriate language for play theme when playing with practitioner/ parent, single peer and/or peer group as assessed during at least 80% of intervals across 2 consecutive probes with practitioner, peer during home peer play session	Picture book reading (can use picture books to guide construction play/theme set up) Construction play (theme set up) or related art/craft activity • Make signs for restaurant, restrooms, and so forth. • Make pretend food. • Make menus. Figurine play • Act out/ implement narratives from restaurant books using toy people, furniture, dishes, blocks, food, materials.	**Sample mands:** I need more blocks to make more tables and chairs. Can I get the food? I need an apron. Can I have that menu? Who do you want to be? Do you want to be the waitress? The customer? The cook? Where should we sit? Do you like pizza? I want a medium pizza with cheese and pepperoni. I want strawberry ice cream for dessert.	**Sample comments:** This is the restaurant. I'm building a restaurant. I'll get my apron and put it on. This customer is ready to order. She wants to order dessert. I'm ordering chocolate and you're having vanilla. You're the mom and I'm the dad. I'm hungry for pizza tonight. I'm going to bake the pizza in the oven.	15-second interval code on topic play and language

(continued)

Embedded Objectives in Play Activity: Restaurant *(continued)*

ITP long-term/ short-term objectives	Theme concepts/ vocabulary		Assessment
	made/drawn during set up. Dress up/role play • Dress up and set up play station— restaurant, kitchen, wait- ress, cus- tomers, and so forth. • Act out/imple- ment narra- tives from restaurant/ cook books. Operationalize "on topic" language Use mands for materials, actions, information re- lated to setting up, organizing, and/ or playing theme. Make comments about (and/or label) materials, his or her own/ partner's play actions related to theme. Count language used to expand/ combine play themes as on topic.	What does the waitress say? Do? What does the customer say/do? What are you doing? Where is my apron? menu? What would you like to order? What are you doing? What are you making? Is the restaurant on this street? Can I have some paper to make a menu? My turn to be the waitress, cus- tomer, cook. You be the wait- ress and I'll be the customer.	First, I'm put- ting on the pepperoni. Here is your coffee. I ordered a medium drink. After dinner, we're having dessert. **Combining play themes:** We have to go grocery shop- ping for the cook. Our restaurant doesn't have any more food. He swallowed a bone. He needs to go to a doctor (doctor activity) The cook burned himself on the oven. Get the first aid kit. The kitchen/ restaurant is on fire. Call 911. (firefighter theme activity)
5. Maintains Topic with Play Actions Blake will maintain a play episode for at least 5 minutes for	Picture book reading (can use picture books to guide construc- tion play/theme set up) Construction play (theme set up) or	**Examples:** • Choose roles and put on apron, hat/coat, and so forth. • Get/use a menu, order	15-second interval code on topic play and language

ITP long-term/ short-term objectives	Theme concepts/ vocabulary	Assessment
5 different themes by performing play actions that are on topic with play theme when playing with practitioner/ parent, single peer and then peer group as assessed during at least 80% of intervals across 2 consecutive probes with practitioner, peer during home peer play session.	related art/craft activity • Make signs for restaurant, restrooms, and so forth. • Make pretend food. • Make menus. Figurine play • Act out/implement narratives from restaurant books using toy people, furniture, dishes, blocks, food, materials made/drawn during set up. • Dress up/role play. • Dress up and set up play station— restaurant, kitchen, waitress, customers, and so forth. • Act out/ implement narratives from restaurant/ cook books. **Operationalize "on-topic" play** • Use materials or producing actions that are related to play theme.	pad, cash register, spatula (look at menu/decide what to order, give/take order, pay cashier). • Draw/color/ paint/build restaurant, kitchen, food, menus, other props to use in play. • Any pretend play action related to play theme—drive to restaurant, sit down at table, give/ look at menu, give/take order, cook/ serve/eat food, pay, clear table, go home, and so forth	
6. **Develop and increase interactive play skills across a variety of topics.**	Figurine play • Act out/implement narratives from restaurant books using toy people, furniture, dishes,		Daily Play Log Video play samples Play Action/Language checklist

(continued)

Embedded Objectives in Play Activity: Restaurant *(continued)*

ITP long-term/ short-term objectives	Theme concepts/ vocabulary	Assessment
Move from single actions to sequenced play actions on a theme with practitioner, peer during home peer play session.	blocks, food, materials made/drawn during set up. • Dress up/role play. • Dress up and set up play station—restaurant, kitchen, waitress, customers, and so forth. • Act out/implement narratives from restaurant/ cook books.	

	Categories	Features	Functions	Assessment
7. Describe/ same/ different	Drinks Desserts Breakfast Foods	Hot Salty Sweet Sticky	Things you drink Things you eat with a spoon Things you cook Things on the menu	Daily Data Sheet—first trial probes

from me. In addition to the behaviors, Blake's speech was also significantly delayed. Prior to his diagnosis he was in speech therapy and was making little progress. When Blake was diagnosed, we were told he may be nonverbal. The thought that I may never be able to have a meaningful conversation with my son was devastating.

We started intensive [Discrete Trial] ABA therapy after Blake's diagnoses. His behavior improved dramatically within the first 6 months, but his speech progressed much slower. He learned how to request items and even began putting some words together; however, he remained extremely delayed in conversational language, and the gap between him and his peers was growing even wider. When Blake was approximately 3½, we began services with the Minnesota Early Autism Project (MEAP). Blake's senior therapist had a background in speech therapy, and the focus of his

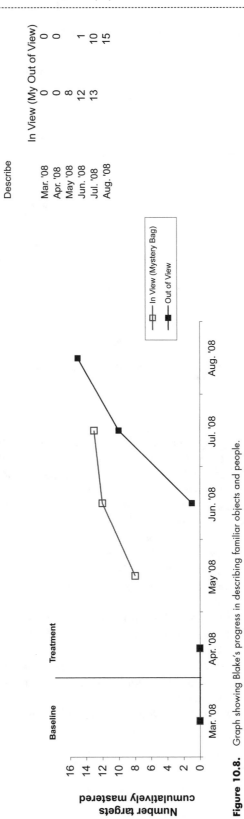

Figure 10.8. Graph showing Blake's progress in describing familiar objects and people.

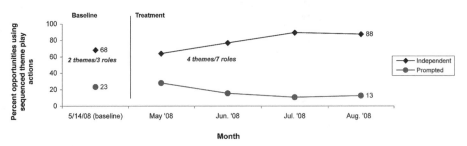

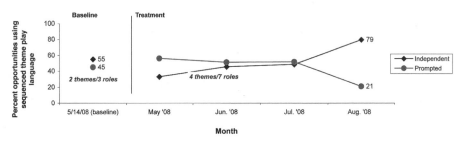

Figure 10.9.   Graph showing Blake's ability to maintain on-topic conversation during spontaneous dress-up play activity while decreasing need for adult prompts.

therapy turned to language and social skills. In our time with MEAP, Blake's language and play skills have exploded. Instead of focusing on Discrete Trial Training, which had been the focus of our last provider, MEAP used a variety of therapies that followed a more natural, environmental approach.

One of the most beneficial programs for Blake was his theme play program. Different themes were introduced to Blake. First he learned about the theme and then he played with the therapist and peers following particular play themes. This helped expand Blake's language and helped teach him to stay on topic.

Blake is currently enrolled in kindergarten with typical peers and is on track to start first grade without any assistance. He is now able to communicate with others and has developed a close relationship with my nephew, who is a year younger than him. They play for hours together and have become best friends. I also no longer have the fear of not being able to communicate with Blake; I'm able to have real conversations with him. Instead of just using words to request what he wants, he has learned to use language to open his world to others. He recently expressed a fear that I would get old and die. Now that he is able to express himself, I can talk to him and calm his fears and anxieties.

Blake's future looks bright, thanks to the therapists at MEAP who thought outside the box and set high goals for him and used creative therapy approaches to accomplish them.

—Emily, mother of Blake

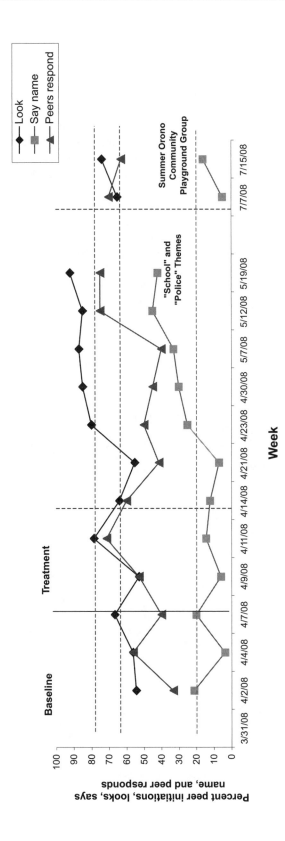

Figure 10.10. Graph showing Blake's learning to accurately recognize what his peers were playing (diamonds), then to comment on their play (squares), and finally to join in their play (triangles).

SUMMARY

Approximately one third to one half of the children with ASDs who have received EIBI services from our program received Blended Behavioral Interventions. Some interventions have included more DTI components, whereas others started with some DTI and made a transition to largely incidental strategies as the children's skills developed. Children who benefit most from DTI intervention tend to have fewer communication and social skills, or some have more significant attention problems. Other children have received half or more of their time in Incidental Teaching Intervention. Studies by Laura Schreibman and colleagues (Schreibman, Stahmer, Barlett, & Dufek, 2009; Sherer & Schreibman, 2005) revealed that children who at baseline engage in toy play and verbal self-stimulation (e.g., echolalia) and who are not socially avoidant did better in PRT, which is consistent with our own observations. Children who have the following characteristics appear to be better candidates for Blended Intervention: 1) low to moderate attention challenges, 2) mild-to-moderate insistence on specific routines, 3) some motor or verbal imitation, 4) intellectual ability in the low average to average range, 5) some joint attention, 6) some speech and gestures, 7) occasional social referencing, and 8) infrequent or occasional motor self-stimulatory behavior. Blended Intervention can be a highly effective form of EIBI for the right child.

REFERENCES

Cooper, J.O., Heron, T.E., & Heward, W.L. (2007). *Applied behavior analysis* (2nd ed.). Upper Saddle River, NJ: Prentice Hall.

DeQuinzio, J.A., Townsend, D.B., Sturmey, P., & Poulson, C.L. (2007). Generalized imitation of facial models by children with autism. *Journal of Applied Behavior Analysis, 40*(4), 755–759.

Hart, B., & Risley, T.R. (1975). Incidental teaching of language in the preschool. *Journal of Applied Behavior Analysis, 8*(4), 411–420.

Jahr, E., Eldevik, S., & Eikeseth, S. (2000). Teaching children with autism to initiate and sustain cooperative play. *Research in Developmental Disabilities, 21*(2), 151–169.

Kaiser, A.P., Yoder, P.J., & Keetz, A. (1992). Evaluating milieu teaching. In S.F. Warren & J. Richlie (Eds.), *Causes and effects in communication and language intervention* (pp. 9–47). Baltimore: Paul H. Brookes Publishing Co.

Koegel, R.I., & Frea, W.D. (1993). Treatment of social behavior in autism through the modification of pivotal social skills. *Journal of Applied Behavior Analysis, 26*(3), 369–377.

Koegel, R.L., & Koegel, L.K. (2006). *Pivotal response treatments for autism: Communication, social, and academic development.* Baltimore: Paul H. Brookes Publishing Co.

Koegel, R.L., Vernon, T.W., & Koegel, L.K. (2009). Improving social initiations in young children with autism using reinforcers with embedded social interactions. *Journal of Autism and Developmental Disorders, 39*(9), 1240–1251.

McGee, G.G., Almeida, M.C., Sulzer-Azaroff, B., & Feldman, R.S. (1992). Promoting reciprocal interactions via peer incidental teaching. *Journal of Applied Behavior Analysis, 25,* 117–126.

McGrath, A.M., Bosch, S., Sullivan, C.L., & Fuqua, R.W. (2003). Training reciprocal social interactions between preschoolers and a child with autism. *Journal of Positive Behavior Interventions, 5,* 47–54.

Miller, J.F., & Chapman, R.S. (1981). The relation between age and mean length of utterance on morphemes. *Journal of Speech and Hearing Research, 24,* 154–161.

Montaigne, M. (1575). *Essays.* (Charles Cotton, Trans.). Retrieved Nov. 8, 2010, from http://oregonstate.edu/instruct/phl302/texts/montaigne/montaigne-essays-1.html#II

Pretti-Frontczak, K., & Bricker, D.D. (2004). *An activity-based approach to early intervention* (3rd ed.). Baltimore: Paul H. Brookes Publishing Co.

Schaefer, C.E., & Kaduson, H.G. (2006). *Contemporary play therapy: Theory, research, and practice.* New York: Guilford Press.

Schrandt, J.A., Townsend, D.B., & Poulson, C.L. (2009). Teaching empathy skills to children with autism. *Journal of Applied Behavior Analysis, 42*(1), 17–32.

Schreibman, L., Stahmer, A.C., Barlett, V., Dufek, S. (2009). Brief report: toward refinement of a predictive behavioral profile for treatment outcome in children with autism. *Research in Autism Spectrum Disorders 3,* 163–172.

Sherer, M.R. & Schreibman, L. (2005) Individual behavioral profiles and predictors of treatment effectiveness for children with autism. *Journal of Consulting and Clinical Psychology, 73,* 525–538.

Sundberg, M.L. (2008). *Verbal behavior milestones assessment and placement program (VB-MAPP).* Concord, CA: Advancements in Verbal Behavior Press.

Wong, C.S., Kasari, C., Freeman, S., & Paparella, T. (2007). The acquisition and generalization of joint attention and symbolic play skills in young children with autism. *Research and Practice for Persons with Severe Disabilities, 32*(2), 101–109.

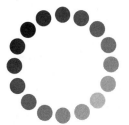 # Postscript

Significant individual differences among children with ASDs challenge us to devise interventions that address that variability (Stahmer, Schreibman, & Cunningham, 2010). From the stories of Jesi to Lilly on one hand and from Patrick to Blake on the other, we have explored the way these individual differences manifest themselves in the day-to-day lives of children with ASDs and their families.

INDIVIDUAL DIFFERENCES AND CHOICE OF INTERVENTION

We have discussed some of the sources of these differences and their implications for intervention for each of the children described in Chapters 7 through 10. If we fail to appreciate these differences, it is difficult to validly assign interventions to individual children. Some of those features are more specific to autism than others, such as limited social understanding and lack of social skills, difficulties with pragmatic language, and fixed interests and repetitive behavior. Other factors are widely distributed throughout the population but interact with these three core features in autism. These include challenges with attention and activity level, anxiety problems, specific speech impairments (such as apraxia of speech), and intellectual functioning level.

The particular blend of interventions that is most appropriate for a given child depends first on the profile of those three core features (see Figure 2.1) and, second, on how those features are moderated by the second group of factors (e.g., anxiety, attention, activity, speech impairment, and intellectual functioning). The Autism Intervention Responsiveness Scale (AIRS,™ Figure 4.1) provides a concrete step toward weighing these factors collectively in predicting the type and combination of interventions that will be most helpful for a child. Though the scale is in a preliminary form, it is a step in the right direction.

OUTCOMES OF COMBINED INTERVENTION APPROACHES

Parents, teachers, and therapists want to know how well a combined intervention approach actually works with young children with autism. Of the first 24 children served by the Minnesota Early Intervention Project from 2006–2010 who participated in from 1 to 3 years of intervention (about 22 hours per week average), 75% have graduated and are currently enrolled in regular education classrooms or are continuing at progressively reduced therapy hours while making the transition to school (Thompson, Barsness, Anderson, & Dropik, manuscript in preparation). About one in five of those children receive some paraprofessional support, two children have been placed in self-contained special education classrooms for students with autism or communication and intellectual disabilities, and two have been placed in early childhood special education classrooms integrated with typically functioning students. One child was discharged due to lack of progress, parents of two children transferred them to other providers (e.g., center-based services), and a fourth moved away. Of those 24 children, 6 received nearly entirely Discrete Trial Intervention, 6 received largely Incidental Intervention, and 12 were provided with a blended combination of Incidental Intervention and DTI. In Blended Interventions, Discrete Trial procedures were often used when introducing a new, especially difficult-to-learn skill, and as soon as the child began showing signs of acquisition, we made the transition to partial Incidental Teaching and eventually entirely Incidental Teaching. Supervisory staff members must be very experienced and well trained for this strategy to work. Hands-on therapists must be competent in using a range of intervention methods. This project suggests it is possible to individualize early behavioral intervention procedures incorporating elements of developmental strategies with behavioral approaches.

MEDICATION COMBINED WITH BEHAVIORAL INTERVENTION

The future holds great promise for preventing and reversing autism symptoms for many children affected with the disability. A promising line of work combines medication to promote brain connectivity with intensive early intervention, possibly as early as 1 year to 18 months of age. Dr. Diane Chugani and her colleagues at Wayne State University have conducted very promising work suggesting that treating children diagnosed with autism at 2 years of age with low doses of a medicine (buspirone) normalizes serotonin in their brain cells, which would otherwise be deficient (Edwards et al., 2006). Proper levels of serotonin are necessary for normal brain connectivity. Dr. Chugani and her colleagues are currently combining EIBI with medication to determine whether these interventions produce a synergistic effect, possibly preventing emergence of autism in some susceptible children (D.C. Chugani, personal communication, June 24, 2010).

Related work suggests it may be possible to treat youngsters with fragile X syndrome with a medication that corrects the balance of proteins that make components of brain synapses (Dolen, Carpenter, Ocain, & Bear, 2010; Penagarikano, Mulle, & Warren, 2007). About one quarter of children with fragile X syndrome also have autism. Together with EIBI, this may make it possible to reduce or eliminate many of the symptoms of autism among children with fragile X and autism.

COMPONENTS OF EARLY INTENSIVE BEHAVIORAL INTERVENTION

The drive to contain educational and health care costs mandates employing the most effective aspects of interventions for specific students or clients. The National Research Council Report called *Educating Children with Autism* (Lord & McGee, 2001) and Reichow and Wolery's (2009) quantitative summary of autism early intervention studies contained two important conclusions: 1) EIBI is highly effective for many children with autism, and 2) which aspects of early behavioral intervention are responsible for these outcomes in subgroups of children is not well understood. We must be able to identify which children benefit most from specific aspects and intensities of intervention. The goal is to identify which aspects of comprehensive early interventions account for the bulk of intervention outcome, so that children optimally benefit from more focused interventions.

Individualizing autism intervention has a promising future, one that may afford the possibility of overcoming or preventing emergence of autism symptoms in susceptible individuals.

REFERENCES

Dolen, G. Carpenter, R.L., Ocain, T.D., Bear, M.F. (2010). Mechanism-based approaches to treating fragile X. *Pharmacology and Therapeutics, 127*(1), 78–93.

Edwards, D.J., Chugani, D.C., Chugani, H.T., Chehab, J., Malin, M., & Aranda, J.V. (2006). Pharmacokinetics of buspirone in autistic children. *Journal of Clinical Pharmacology, 46,* 508–514.

Lord., C., & McGee, J.P. (Eds.). (2001). *Educating children with autism.* Washington, DC: National Academies Press.

Penagarikano, O., Mulle, J.G., & Warren. S.T. (2007).The pathophysicology of fragile X syndrome. *Annual Review of Genomics and Human Genetics, 8,* 109–129.

Reichow, B., & Wolery, M. (2009). Comprehensive synthesis of early intensive behavioral interventions for young children with autism based on the UCLA young autism project model. *Journal of Autism and Developmental Disorders, 39*(1), 23–41.

Stahmer, A.C., Schreibman, L., & Cunningham, A.B. (2010). Toward a technology of treatment individualization in autism spectrum disorders. *Brain Research,* 2010 September 18. EPub Ahead of Print. PMID: 20858466.

Thompson, T. (2010, June). *Can we all get along? Toward blended autism interventions.* Career Scientist Award Speech, Experimental Analysis of Human Behavior SIG, Association for Behavior Analysis International Annual Conference, San Antonio, Texas.

Thompson, T., Barsness, L., Anderson, C., Burggraff, B., & Dropik, P. (in preparation) *Individualized Intensive Early Behavioral Intervention for young children with autism: Predictors of type of treatment and outcomes.*

Index

Page numbers followed by *f* indicate figures.